Most of the articles, letters, and resources in this book appeared originally in *Mothering* Magazine between 1979 and 1997.

Published by *Mothering* Magazine, Inc.
PO Box 1690
Santa Fe, New Mexico 87504
Printed in the United States of America

ISBN:0-914257-17-X

Vaccination
The Issue of Our Times

A Selection of Articles, Letters, and
Resources
1979–1997

Edited by Peggy O'Mara

CONTENTS

INTRODUCTION: YOUR CHOICE.................................6
PEGGY O'MARA

A SHORT HISTORY OF VACCINATION 9
FREDERICK HODGES

THE EXPERTS' FORUM 24
VACCINATION RISKS AND BENEFITS CHARTS 58
UNDERSTANDING THE POLIO VACCINE 64
ANNE MONTGOMERY

WEIGHING THE FACTS ABOUT PERTUSSIS.......................68
JAY GORDON

THE NEW DTP: DTAP 71
ANNE MONTGOMERY

TO VACCINATE OR NOT? A GUIDE FOR MAKING A CHOICE 72
MIRANDA CASTRO

THE VACCINATIONS 74
THE MMR VACCINE 76
LYNNE MCTAGGART

THE CHICKENPOX VACCINE 86
MARYANN NAPOLI

CONSIDERING VARICELLA.....................................89
ANNE MONTGOMERY

CHICKENPOX: LIVE AND LET LIVE 90
JAY GORDON

PERTUSSIS (WHOOPING COUGH) 91
CAROL MILLER

VACCINATIONS...94
MAGDA KRANCE

INFORMED CONSENT 98
VACCINE POLICY: A SHOT AT YOUR RIGHTS 100
PEGGY CYPHER

ADVERSE EFFECTS OF CHILDHOOD VACCINES.....................104
THE INSTITUTE OF MEDICINE

Contents

VACCINATION PRECAUTIONS 108
VICKI GILES

VACCINATIONS AND INFORMED CHOICE............................112
MAGDA KRANCE

IMMUNIZATIONS AND INFORMED CONSENT 122
CAROL MILLER

CONSTITUTIONAL RIGHTS AND IMMUNIZATION 129
CAROL MILLER

PHILOSOPHICAL QUESTIONS 132
IMMUNIZATIONS: THE OTHER SIDE 134
RICHARD MOSKOWITZ

BRINGING VACCINES INTO PERSPECTIVE 146
HAROLD E. BUTTRAM AND JOHN CHRISS HOFFMAN

UNVACCINATED CHILDREN 158
RICHARD MOSKOWITZ

VACCINATION: A SACRAMENT OF MODERN MEDICINE 168
RICHARD MOSKOWITZ

THE READERS' DIALOGUE 1979–1997.....................178
LETTERS

GOOD NEWS 246
1987–1997

CHILDHOOD DISEASES 260
WHOOPING COUGH 262
ANNA JOYCE

HELPFUL INFORMATION 266
ANNA JOYCE

NATURAL REMEDIES FOR CHILDHOOD DISEASES 268
MIRANDA CASTRO

AROMATHERAPY AND CHILDHOOD DISEASES 282
CHRISTA OBUCHOWSKI

RESOURCES 286

STATE EXEMPTIONS 306

Introduction: Your Choice

By Peggy O'Mara

We present the information in this book in the spirit of informed consent. The vaccination decision is one of the most difficult and emotionally charged decisions that parents must make.

When *Mothering* first covered the down side of vaccinations in 1979, we did so because vaccinations was the most popular topic in our letters section. It was a popular topic because our original readers, natural living pioneers, were theoretically opposed to invasive practices, but needed information and support to make difficult, complex, and highly personal vaccination decisions.

The material in this book was originally published between 1979 and 1997. The older articles give an overview of the evolution of the vaccination debate. Newer articles contain current research, opinions, and extensive updated resources.

Parents are under tremendous pressure to vaccinate. And, indeed, vaccinations are effective. Medical professionals are under tremendous pressure to ensure vaccine compliance at the same time that consumers' questions are on the rise. We need tolerance of each other's values and biases.

Some of the more than 200 viral and bacterial vaccines currently being created by federal health agencies and vaccines manufacturers include:

Chlamydia

Cholera

Cytomegalovirus

Dengue virus

E. coli

Epstein-Barr virus

Gonorrhea

Group A Streptococcus

Group B Streptococcus

Hepatitis C virus

Hepatitis D virus

Hepatitis E virus

Herpes simplex virus types 1 and 2

HIV-1 (44 different kinds)

HIV-2 (7 different kinds)

Human papillomavirus

Influenza virus (7 different kinds)
Japanese B encephalitis virus
Legionella Pneumophila
Mycoplasma pneumoniae
Meningitis A,B, and C
Parainfluenza virus
Respiratory syncytial virus
Rotavirus (diarrhea)
Salmonella typhi
Shigella
Streptococcus pneumoniae
Toxoplasma gondii
Tuberculosis
No information is available on plans for use or distribution of these vaccinations.

Vaccine development has become big business. Worldwide revenues of nearly $3 billion are expected to more than double to $7 billion over the next five years as more vaccines are developed. Vaccine industry revenues are estimated at more than $1 billion a year in the US alone. This is up from $500 million in 1990, a 200 percent increase over six years. The cost to fully immunize a child has risen from $107 in 1986 to $367 in 1996, a 243 percent increase over ten years.

In 1954, Bernice Eddy, a doctor of bacteriology, discovered live monkey viruses in supposedly inactivated polio vaccines developed by Dr. Jonas Salk. One of these viruses, SV40, is a simian virus. Simians, or monkeys, are used in scientific experimentation and development in viral, cancer, and vaccine research and have a high incidence of viruses, many of which are harmless.

Between 1959 and 1965, research of pregnant women showed the incidence of brain tumors in children of Salk vaccinated mothers to be 13 times greater than children of mothers who hadn't received the Salk vaccine. German scientists have found evidence of SV40 in 30 out of 110 brain tumors. Brain tumors have increased 30 percent in the US over the last 20 years.

When the National Academy of Science's Institute of Medicine attempted to verify particular vaccine reactions, they found a dearth of studies on vaccine reactions in general. The National Institutes of

Health spends approximately $415 million a year promoting vaccines and new vaccine research, and little if any of this funding is allocated to studying vaccine reactions. It is difficult to study the long-term effects of vaccines while vaccination is compulsory and as long as so little research funding is directed at such studies.

As parents, we are increasingly asked to vaccinate our children against diseases that we seldom see and about which we are not worried. We wonder why hepatitis B is given to babies when it is a sexually transmitted disease. The three recommended doses of hepatitis B vaccinations costs $40 or more. The duration of protection is unknown, and booster shot requirements are undefined. We wonder why more reactive vaccines stay on the market when safer vaccines are available. And we wonder if there are contaminants in vaccines.

As parents, we want our concerns taken seriously. The public health crusade to eradicate disease does so sometimes at the expense of our children. This is not acceptable to us as parents, nor should it be acceptable in a civilized society.

It is unethical in a time of so many questions about vaccinations or in any time to deny philosophical exemptions. It is unjust to ask parents to become medical experts in order to protect their children. And it is immoral to risk the health of even one child in order to save the lives of many.

A Short History of Vaccination
By Frederick Hodges

Frederick Hodges is an historian at the Wellcome Unit for the History of Medicine at Oxford University. Hodges received his undergraduate degree at the University of California at Berkeley. He has been published in the British Medical Journal, *the* Journal of Urology, *the* Journal of Pediatrics, Urology, *and other leading international medical journals. He has also contributed a historical chapter to* Sexual Mutilations: A Human Tragedy *(New York: Plenum Press, 1997), edited by George C. Denniston, MD, and Marilyn Fayre Milos, RN.*

Introduction

The history of vaccination represents one of the great epics of modern medicine. The search for vaccines led incidentally to the discoveries of the germ theory of disease and the immune system.

Smallpox

Smallpox was a native Asiatic disease that spread to Europe because of the opening of trade routes to Asia and Africa. As a result of the unsanitary living conditions created by the Industrial Revolution in Europe, this rare disease became a leading killer. Older European towns and cities, which had no sewage disposal systems or running water, suddenly swelled with overworked, undernourished, underpaid, uneducated, unwashed masses packed into abominably filthy, unventilated, unheated tenements and hovels by night and crowded into airless and sunless factories by day. These conditions allowed previously rare microbial infections such as smallpox to flourish into raging epidemics. Even though 75 percent of those who contracted smallpox survived, 15 million Europeans alone died of smallpox every 25 years.

In its native Oriental realms, the true nature of smallpox was no better understood by its victims than in Europe. What centuries of observation and acquired folk wisdom had led Orientals and Africans to understand was that a smallpox infection survivor became immune to future infections. They also understood that smallpox was infectious; that is, that an infected healthy person could transmit it to a previously uninfected person.

In antiquity, Chinese doctors used these observations to formulate and execute a plan of action: They dried and pulverized smallpox scabs and blew them into the noses of healthy individuals through special bone inoculation tubes. The desired result was usually a mild case of smallpox, which, in effect, immunized the patient against any severe future cases. In Asia Minor and Africa, similar methods of immunization were used. In some cultures, healthy people were induced to swallow the scabs or pus of infected persons. In others, native healers opened veins or scratched healthy skin with needles and rubbed infected pus into the wounds.

In the American colonies, smallpox was no less a scourge than in Europe. African slaves taught their colonial masters the ancient technique of inoculation. The Boston clergyman Cotton Mather learned this technique from the African Onesimos, who was one of his slaves. In 1721, Mather persuaded physician Zabdiel Boylston to use the African method of smallpox inoculation to ward off a current outbreak.

This technique was given the name variolation from the Latinate word for smallpox, *variola*. After smallpox decimated the rebel colonial troops besieging Quebec, George Washington ordered the variolation of the entire Continental Army, thereby ensuring the victory of the American Revolutionary forces over the unvariolated British troops. Still, variolation had a death rate of 1 in 300, leading some colonies, such as Virginia, to outlaw its use.

In 1722, after some of the grandchildren of the British royal family were variolated, noble and upper-class families routinely variolated their children. British physicians and apothecaries transformed variolation into a lengthy and costly procedure, one whose necessity was insisted upon, and one that generated enormous profits for its practitioners. Inoculation hospitals, to which upper-class boarding school boys were routinely sent, were actually barns or stables where the boys were kept tied together for six weeks in conditions of filth and degradation. The boys were regularly bled, purged, starved, and dosed with noxious medicines, ostensibly to purify their blood. After this, they were inoculated with pus from smallpox victims pressed into an open wound created by a knife tip. The boys were then put back into the barn, where, after a week, the lucky ones developed only a mild case of smallpox, complete with fever, vomiting, and diarrhea. Those who survived were not allowed to leave the barn until their smallpox scars had fallen off. Such private inoculation hospitals sprang up all over England.

One man who was forced to endure the unnecessary torments

of the inoculation hospital as a boy was Edward Jenner (1749–1823), a young country doctor from Berkeley, Gloucestershire. The country folk of this shire, whose poverty protected them from the inoculation hospitals, had noticed that dairymaids who had contracted the innocuous disease of cowpox from cows were subsequently immune to smallpox. Jenner was intrigued by this possibility, but when he brought it before his professional colleagues, he was roundly attacked and threatened with expulsion from the county medical society.

On May 14, 1796, Jenner treated a Gloucestershire dairymaid, Sarah Nelmes, for sores on her fingers caused by cowpox she had contracted from a cow's infected utters. Jenner drew some lymph from Sarah Nelmes's cowpox pustules and set it aside. Later that same day, he inoculated the cowpox lymph into a needle scratch on the arm of eight-year-old James Phipps. As expected, young James developed a mild case of cowpox. On July 1, Jenner took the bold step of inoculating James with pus taken from a person with true smallpox. James had no reaction. A few weeks later, Jenner inoculated James again with another dose of smallpox pustular matter taken from yet another smallpox patient. Again, the boy remained unaffected.

Without understanding the scientific basis for his results, Jenner had nevertheless established scientifically that cowpox inoculation rendered the subject immune to smallpox. To commemorate the bovine role in this procedure, Jenner named it "vaccination," from the Latin word *vaccinus*, "relating to cows."

Jenner repeated the vaccination procedure on various local people. In 1798, he self-published his experimental results in a little book entitled *An Inquiry into the Causes and Effects of the Variolae Vaccinae*, in which he urged the universal use of his cowpox vaccine to rid the world of the deadly scourge of smallpox. In so doing, Jenner made many powerful enemies.

The most powerful of these was the Reverend Thomas Robert Malthus. Malthus, like his religious predecessor, Reverend Joseph Townsend, condemned any efforts to prevent pestilential diseases as a direct affront to "God's scheme of things." Smallpox and other such plagues were, according to Townsend and Malthus, the Christian God's tools for regulating the population and punishing those wicked enough to have been born poor. These men and their followers additionally opposed any efforts to improve sanitation and housing conditions in urban centers.

Jenner was also opposed and attacked as a charlatan by prominent and powerful members of the British medical profession, many of whom had a vested interest in the highly lucrative inoculation hospital scam. By nature a trusting man, Jenner, while on a mission to London to seek support for vaccination, entrusted some inoculant to a Dr. William Woodville, who, posing as a supporter, actually ran an inoculation hospital. Woodville deliberately and secretly contaminated the cowpox vaccine with live smallpox virus in an attempt to prove that Jenner's vaccine was dangerously ineffective. Even after Jenner's death in 1823, vaccination opponents, most of whom had vested interests in the inoculation hospitals, or who had religious and commercial interests in the continuation of poverty and human misery, published in reputable medical journals bogus accounts of cowpox-vaccinated people developing bovine facial features.

Despite the proven effectiveness and cheapness of Jenner's vaccine and its promise of freeing all humans, both rich and poor, from the threat of smallpox, Malthus and his supporters opposed and killed almost all legislation providing for public vaccination. Though the public demanded the passage of such bills, those that passed were so weakened or devoid of necessary funding as to be ineffective and unenforceable.

In contrast to the British government's inability to protect its British subjects, other European nations were quick to recognize the value of Jenner's vaccine. Beginning in the first decade of the 19th century, Bavaria, Denmark, Sweden, Würtemberg, Prussia, Romania, Hungary, and Serbia, in succession, all made universal vaccination available and immediately enjoyed its benefits.

Despite the campaign of scare tactics and chicanery from a hostile medical profession, the value of Jenner's vaccine proved itself in time. In 1800, the vaccine was used successfully in Vienna to combat a smallpox epidemic. The British Army, remembering the lessons of the American Revolution and succumbing less to political intrigue from religious pressure groups, adopted a policy of routine vaccination of the military population. The next year, the admiralty had the entire British fleet vaccinated and presented Jenner with a special gold medal for his service to mankind. In 1804, Napoleon ordered the entire French Army vaccinated and, not to be outdone by the English, presented Jenner with a somewhat more elaborate gold medal.

After Jenner's death, Parliament passed an 1835 bill making infant vaccination compulsory in England and Wales, and, ten years later, passed a companion act mandating vaccination in Scotland and Ireland. Various other supporting acts were passed, but, thanks to the Malthusians, none was properly funded or implemented. As a result, Britain was devastated by the great smallpox pandemic from 1870 to 1875. In 1871, smallpox deaths reached 2,432 per million in London alone.

Through the agency of one of Jenner's American supporters, Dr. Benjamin Waterhouse, president Thomas Jefferson vaccinated his entire family, which amounted to more than 70 persons. Jefferson took great interest in vaccination and, in 1801, wrote Jenner a letter of praise.

In the US, from 1820 to 1875, smallpox epidemics hit every major city, all of which were crowded and filthy, and lacked sewage disposal systems and clean water. The sanitary movement in America, led by reformers such as Sylvester Graham and Lemuel Shattuck, did much to improve the infrastructure of American cities and to slow the spread of contagious diseases such as smallpox. Because of Shattuck and his supporters' efforts, American municipalities slowly adopted programs of universal vaccination. Still, these programs' implementation was inadequate at best. During the same era, European nations such as Germany and Sweden had almost completely eradicated the disease, while the US still had the highest rate of smallpox deaths of any Western nation until the mid-20th century.

Vaccination, however, was not always safe. Human arm-to-arm transfers of cowpox virus could allow the passing of whatever microbial diseases the donor incidentally may have had. Transmission of syphilis, leprosy, hepatitis, and other usually fatal diseases through human arm-to-arm transfers was common. In the era prior to the acceptance and understanding of the germ theory of disease, such accidental transmissions of diseases were blamed on vaccination in general, rather than on the improper *mode* of vaccination.

Acting rationally, the New York City Board of Health ceased human arm-to-arm transfers. It then opened a vaccine farm in 1876 to produce good vaccine from clean calves. Still, not all vaccines were safe. Unscrupulous or criminally negligent manufacturers sold vaccines that were often as ineffective as they were contaminated with dangerous and deadly microbes such as tetanus (lockjaw) acquired from sick cows or unsanitary manufacturing practices.

LOUIS PASTEUR AND THE GERM THEORY OF DISEASE

While not the first to state it, the French chemist Louis Pasteur (1822–1895) was one of the first to fully understand the implications of the germ theory of disease and was certainly one of its most ardent defenders. In 1878, in order to concretely prove that specific bacteria caused specific diseases, Pasteur devoted his research to chicken cholera. Dr. H. Toussaint had already isolated a bacterium (now called *Pasteurella multocida*) in the fluids of chickens with chicken cholera but could not culture the organism. Pasteur found a way to culture the organism and, on feeding chickens a single drop of it, induced cholera.

In the summer of 1879, Pasteur and his assistants went on vacation, leaving a batch of chicken cholera culture in the laboratory refrigerator. Upon his return several months later, Pasteur inoculated healthy chickens with the aged culture. To his surprise, the aged culture did not produce disease in the chickens. Using a fresh batch of virulent cholera culture, he then inoculated two groups of chickens: a group of previously uninoculated chickens and the original group that had remained unaffected by the aged culture inoculation. Nearly all the previously inoculated chickens remained healthy, while the new chickens developed chicken cholera. Pasteur described this age-dependent weakening process as "attenuation." Quickly realizing the potential of his discovery, Pasteur honored Jenner by naming his chicken-immunizing agent "vaccine," though it had nothing to do with cows.

Pasteur next turned his attention to the sheep disease anthrax. Through experimentation, he learned that heat treatment could attenuate the anthrax bacilli, producing an effective "vaccine."

Pasteur also developed a vaccine against rabies, even though he never isolated or identified its causal agent. Rabies, unlike cholera or anthrax, is caused by a virus, and viruses would remain invisible to science until the invention of the electron microscope after World War II. Normally a vaccine would be ineffective against a microbial infection, but Pasteur noted that rabies had a long incubation period before symptoms appeared. His experiments with dogs established the effectiveness of his new rabies "vaccine."

Pasteur had always refused to experiment on humans, but in 1885, a local doctor who had followed his activities brought him a nine-year-old Alsatian schoolboy who had been bitten by a rabid dog. Pasteur agreed to the doctor's entreaty to inject the boy with the experimental curative vaccine. During the virus' incubation period, Pasteur treated him with his series of age-graded inoculations, and, when the boy remained free of rabies, Pasteur became an instant celebrity. The French government set up the new Pasteur Institute and foreign branches in which Pasteur could train the most promising scientific minds.

THE SEARCH FOR NEW VACCINES

Following Pasteur's demonstration that attenuation of pathogenic microbes transformed some pathogens into vaccines, the international scientific community rushed to identify and convert into vaccines the leading causes of death in the industrial world: tuberculosis, pneumonia, cholera, dysentery, diphtheria, meningitis, influenza, typhoid, childbed fever, and sexually transmitted diseases. Corrupt pharmaceutical companies quickly started producing vaccines scientifically "proven" to prevent all these diseases and more. Medical journals rushed into print successful accounts of the discovery of "miracle" vaccines for tuberculosis, syphilis, and other such diseases. American medical journals also started carrying advertisements for and receiving enticing funds from pharmaceutical companies selling such vaccines. Most, if not all, of these vaccines were worthless; many were even harmful. And though they were published in the leading medical journals, supporting studies were bogus. But then, as now, it was difficult for many to accept that pharmaceutical companies could be guilty of chicanery.

Another factor that muddied the waters of scientific advancement was the fierce and pointless competition that existed among the various medical systems available to American healthcare consumers. Homeopathists, who in the 19th century provided a significant proportion of the nation's health care, enthusiastically endorsed vaccination programs. Often for no other reason than this, many regular physicians took a defensive stand against vaccination. Conveniently ignoring Pasteur's undeniable successes, they bolstered their positions by pointing to the worthless, even harmful vaccines produced by clandestinely dishonest manufacturers.

All of the contagious diseases for which science sought vaccines had fertile breeding ground in the filthy, overcrowded, poverty-stricken cites of the Western world and were, in a sense, caused by these industry-generated conditions. Efforts to improve living conditions of urban-dwelling Americans may very well have as effectively slowed the spread of communicable diseases as did the vaccines and therapies the scientific world simultaneously turned out.

For example, pneumonia at the turn of the century was the leading cause of death in the world and actually killed more Panama Canal workers than either yellow fever or malaria. It was largely eradicated due to the intelligence of William C. Gorgas (1854–1920), then surgeon general of the US Army. Gorgas simply recommended that the canal workers' pay be doubled. Workers then could move out of their overcrowded, unventilated, pestilential barracks and into private accommodations where they could afford to grow or purchase nourishing food.

Similarly, during World War I, specifically in the first months of 1918, more American soldiers died in American military training camps of pneumonia resulting from influenza than were killed in battle in Europe. The crowding of soldiers into unventilated barracks led to epidemics of pneumonia, measles, mumps, meningitis, and other communicable diseases. After an inspection of US military training camps in response to reports of increasing cases of and deaths from infectious diseases, Gorgas testified before the Senate Military Affairs Committee in January 1918 that these senseless deaths could be prevented simply by eliminating overcrowding in military barracks.

Rather than accepting Gorgas's urgent medical recommendations and making US military bases safe for millions of young American men, President Woodrow Wilson in effect fired Gorgas that October. The result was the needless and preventable deaths of more than a half-million Americans. The significance of this death rate is evident when compared with the 53,000 servicemen killed in battle.

In addition to the efforts to improve American living conditions, the quest for a pneumonia vaccine continued. For decades, European and American scientists searched for the answer, but it remained illusive because it was not understood that pneumonia can be caused by at least 83 types of *pneumococci*. Vaccines developed to prevent one type of *pneumococci* were ineffective against all the others.

In 1927, two scientists working at the Robert Koch Institute for Infectious Diseases in Berlin, Wolfgang Casper and Oscar Schiemann, discovered by accident an effective vaccine against pneumonia. They had been conducting experiments on the toxicity of the pneumococcal capsules and measuring the lethalness of various doses of *pneumococci*. This miracle of scientific achievement was, however, destined to be short-lived. With the development of sulfa drugs in 1938 and antibiotics after World War II, pneumonia could be more cheaply treated than prevented. The manufacture of pneumonia vaccines all but ceased.

THE DISCOVERY OF THE VIRUS

Edward Jenner was completely unaware that the agents of smallpox and cowpox were viruses. He had no idea that bacteria existed, either. Yet even without any understanding of the germ theory of disease, of the immune system, or of bacteriology, virology, cell theory, of blood chemistry, he had discovered an effective smallpox vaccine. Pasteur, likewise, was unaware of the existence of viruses. He assumed that his inability to detect the bacterial agent for diseases such as rabies and smallpox was due to the extreme smallness of the bacteria he concluded must be present. Pasteur incorrectly theorized that cowpox was an attenuation of smallpox and that the attenuation was produced by the microbe having passed through the cow's body. This incorrect explanation for Jenner's vaccine nevertheless led him to develop a true rabies vaccine by imitating the animal attenuation process.

Pasteur had passed virulent rabies virus from the saliva of rabid dogs through the brain and spinal columns of rabbits. What emerged was a serum capable of stimulating the body of another animal to produce antibodies against the virus without permitting the virus to produce disease. Other scientists observed that body fluids drawn from patients (or experimental animals) suffering from viral infections would still inoculate healthy animals with the same viral infection even after the fluid had been passed through the most minute bacterial filters. Scientists called these filterable "bacteria" *viruses* (from the Latin word for "poison") because they mistakenly believed that the disease agent was a bacteria-produced toxin rather than the bacteria themselves.

Max Theiler (1899–1972), of the Rockefeller Institute, created an effective yellow fever vaccine in 1936 by repeating Pasteur's technique of attenuating what would decades later be identified as viruses by passing them through the brain tissues of animals—in this case mice. With the advent of the German-designed electron microscope, these submicroscopic, filterable "bacterial" toxins were found to be an entirely new class of microbe: the virus.

THE CONQUEST OF POLIO

Apart from the fraudulent polio vaccines that proliferated around the turn of the century, many of the world's top scientists worked for decades to discover the exact nature of polio and a vaccine against it. In 1908, Viennese scientist Karl Landsteiner (1868–1943) proved that polio was a transmissible infectious "viral" disease not a bacterial disease by injecting into a monkey sterile filtrates from the spinal cord tissue of a child who had died of polio. In 1911, Swedish scientists Carl Kling (1887–1967), Alfred Pettersson, and Wilhelm Wernstedt correctly determined that polio invades the gastrointestinal tract through food and water. It usually causes only a mild, generally unnoticeable infection, giving the body time to develop natural immunity to subsequent polio infections, then passes out of the body. Polio was thus a very common part of the environment, which only rarely spread to the central nervous system and caused paralysis in nonimmune, susceptible children and, even more rarely, adults.

Unfortunately, America ignored Kling's correct findings; the false hypothesis of Rockefeller Institute doctors Simon Flexner and Paul Lewis was believed instead. Flexner and Lewis held that polio was a respiratory virus that entered the body through the nose and from there directly invaded the brain and spinal cord. This tragic error delayed scientific advancement and rational social sanitation policy for decades, costing millions of people their lives and health. Another false theory, advanced in 1912, was that polio was an insect-borne disease transmitted by the common stable fly. This attractive theory gained more converts than the more prosaic but correct Swedish discovery.

Despite these setbacks, real progress was made with time. In 1934, Maurice Brodie (1903–1939) and William H. Park (1863–1939), who had earlier developed an effective diphtheria vaccine, pioneered a formalin-inactivated, or killed-virus poliovirus vaccine. In the same year, Dr. John A. Kolmer, of the Dermatological Research Laboratory in Philadelphia, announced the development of a chemically attenuated live poliovirus vaccine. The following year, 10,000 children were injected with the Park-Brodie vaccine and 12,000 children with the Kolmer vaccine. Park, Brodie, and Kolmer reported that their polio vaccines were successful, but doctors around the country reported that children vaccinated with these vaccines had contracted paralytic polio, and some children had died. Tragically, these men, like most American scientists, had dogmatically insisted that only one strain of polio virus existed. They arrogantly dismissed a 1931 study by two Australian doctors, Macfarlane Burnett and Jan Macnamara, who had uncovered at least two strains of polio virus. This arrogance cost Brodie, Park, and Kolmer their careers.

It is quite possible that the Park-Brodie and Kolmer vaccines were effective against one type of polio virus and that the postvaccinal cases and deaths were caused by a rarer type. Starting in 1949, Dr. David Bodian, of Johns Hopkins, working with the National Foundation for Infantile Paralysis (the March of Dimes), eventually identified more than 200 strains of polio virus, which fell into three main categories.

In 1949, while working on a mumps vaccine at Children's Hospital in Boston, John F. Enders, Frederick Robbins, and Thomas Weller accidentally discovered that the poliovirus was not, despite contrary American medical dogma, limited to neural tissues. They found, as the Swedish had, that it thrived in the gastrointestinal tract and in human tissue cultures.

From 1952 to 1954, thanks to the technical advances of the Enders group, Dr. Jonas Salk, of the University of Pittsburgh, revised the Park-Brodie formalin-inactivated polio vaccine, this time containing the Type I, II, and III strains he had grown in monkey kidney tissue cultures. Salk's vaccine worked well in clinical trials until April 1955, when reports of vaccine-associated poliomyelitis started. Of the 204 cases that occurred, 79 were in vaccinated children, 105 were among vaccinated children's family members, and 20 were among contacts in the community. Three-quarters of the cases were paralytic poliomyelitis, and 11 people died. Investigation revealed that in seven lots of vaccine manufactured by Cutter Laboratories of

Berkeley, California, the poliovirus had not been killed. No other problems were associated with the Salk killed-virus vaccine, and Denmark, Sweden, and Finland entirely eliminated the virus using the Salk vaccine alone.

In 1954, the National Foundation for Infantile Paralysis gave Dr. Albert Sabin a grant to develop a live poliovirus vaccine. Over the next decade, Sabin had his live virus vaccine tested internationally on millions. Sabin realized that the advantage of a live virus vaccine is that it is taken orally and thus more closely resembles the natural infection route. The gastrointestinal mucosa of the upper gastrointestinal tract immediately begins producing alpha globulin antibodies to the virus. The Salk killed-virus vaccine is injected intramuscularly, taking up to 46 hours before it slowly migrates from the muscles into the circulatory system. The orally administered Sabin vaccine requires only one dose, whereas the Salk intramuscularly injected formalin-killed vaccine requires three injected doses. In March 1962, the Sabin trivalent (containing Types I, II, and III) was licensed and used to immunize millions of American adults and children. While both vaccines are equally effective, the Sabin vaccine has almost completely superseded the Salk vaccine in the US.

MEASLES, MUMPS, AND RUBELLA

Measles appears to have arrived in Europe from Asia at approximately the same time and by the same routes as smallpox, whose symptoms it closely replicates. Like most other infectious diseases, measles is associated with overcrowding, poverty, and unsanitary living conditions. While almost unknown today in industrial countries with strong vaccination programs, it was once a major American scourge, killing more children than any other infectious disease.

Measles was also closely associated with military training camps. The effect of massing together conscripts from every part of the country exposed previously unexposed, and thus unimmune, males to incapacitating microbial infections. As with smallpox, early preventative efforts took the form of "variolation." Measles, however, could not be inoculated using pus. Instead, direct inoculation was only possible by using an infected person's blood. In 1911, after injecting a monkey with cell-free blood filtrate from a measles patient, American scientists established that measles was, in fact, what would later be called a virus. An American worker developed an unsuccessful vaccine in 1938 at the Pasteur Institute in Paris, but the first successful vaccine (the Edmonston live measles virus vaccine) was not licensed for US use until 1963.

Rubella (German measles) was traditionally a more common childhood disease than measles. In most children, rubella has only mild symptoms and confers lifelong immunity against its recurrence. In 1938, Japanese doctors proved that rubella was a virus rather than a bacterium, but little effort was made to develop a vaccine because the disease was relatively innocuous. Two years later, however, an Australian rubella epidemic showed doctors that pregnant women who contracted the disease often had babies with serious birth defects. From 1963 to 1964, the US suffered the worst rubella epidemic in its history, in which at least 20,000 children were born severely brain damaged. Countless other birth defects may have resulted, but because rubella was not then a notifiable disease, no records exist to confirm this. In 1966, Drs. Paul Parkman, Harry Meyer, Jr., and Theodore C. Panos, of the Federal Bureau of Biologics, developed an attenuated live rubella virus vaccine.

Mumps is a viral disease that is usually very mild but can, in rare cases, cause sterility in males, deafness, pancreatitis, and severe brain encephalitis leading to brain damage and mental retardation. The first mumps vaccine was developed by John F. Enders and Joseph Stokes, Jr., for armed forces use during World War II. Though this vaccine had only short-term effectiveness, the Soviet Union simultaneously developed a live-virus vaccine conferring lifelong immunity, which was used on millions of Soviet children. Dr. Maurice Hilleman and Eugene Buynack developed a live-virus vaccine attenuated through chick embryo cultures. The Hilleman mumps vaccine was licensed in January 1968.

HEPATITIS B

Hepatitis B is a blood-borne virus, which, at least in the US, is a common sexually transmitted disease among intravenous drug users and urban homosexuals. Unlike other communicable viruses, it is not transmissible through the air or through casual contact. It therefore poses a potential threat only for those who deliberately place themselves in risky situations. Despite these epidemiological facts, efforts have been made since the 1960s to develop a vaccine against it.

In 1961, Dr. Saul Krugman, of New York University, discovered that the hepatitis B virus could be attenuated simply by boiling it in water for one minute. Nine years later, Maurice Hilleman and his Merck Institute colleagues developed the hepatitis B vaccine based on the work of Krugman and others. Vaccine trials began in 1978 among the New York City homosexual population, and it was proven 92.3 percent effective. The drug industry-led effort to require hepatitis B vaccine for all American children is scientifically and epidemiologically insupportable. This situation has been viewed with great cynicism by the American public and has greatly eroded the public's confidence in the medical profession and in vaccination in general.

THE PRESENT STATUS OF VACCINATION

Vaccines of various degrees of effectiveness and harmfulness have been developed for other contagious diseases such as hepatitis A, chickenpox, influenza, and the common cold. Efforts to find vaccines for certain microbial infections such as syphilis and gonorrhea have been halted by the discovery of antibiotics, which make it more economical to treat certain diseases—especially those that are contracted deliberately rather than accidentally—instead of immunizing everyone against them.

The wide selection of successful vaccines against deadly—or at the very least unpleasant—diseases is a testament to the proven effectiveness of some vaccines. For instance, it is completely due to Jenner's vaccine that smallpox was entirely eliminated from the planet, and officially declared to be so by the World Health Organization in 1977. Regardless of the controversy over valid human rights questions raised by compulsory vaccination policies, vaccination remains one of many scientifically proven tools to eliminate airborne contagious diseases and improve human life.

BIBLIOGRAPHY

Baxby, Derrick. *Jenner's Smallpox Vaccine: The Riddle of Vaccinia Virus and Its Origin.* London: Heinemann Educational Books, 1981.

Chase, Allan. *Magic Shots.* New York: William Morrow, 1982.

Cohen, Bernard, ed. *Cotton Mather and American Science and Medicine: With Studies and Documents Concerning the Introduction of Inoculation or Variolation.* New York: Arno Press, 1980.

Cohen, Bernard, ed. *The Life and Scientific and Medical Career of*

Benjamin Waterhouse: With Some Account of the Introduction of Vaccination in America. New York: Arno Press, 1980.

Fisher, Richard B. *Edward Jenner, 1749–1823*. London: AndreDeutsch, 1991.

Geison, Gerald L. *The Private Science of Louis Pasteur*. Princeton, NJ: Princeton University Press, 1995.

Jenner, Edward. *Letters of Edward Jenner, and Other Documents Concerning the Early History of Vaccination*. Genevieve Miller, ed. Baltimore, MD: Johns Hopkins University Press, 1983.

Muraskin, William A. *The War Against Hepatitis B: A History of the International Task Force on Hepatitis B Immunization*. Philadelphia: University of Pennsylvania Press, 1995.

Needham, Joseph. *China and the Origins of Immunology*. Hong Kong: Centre of Asian Studies, University of Hong Kong, 1980.

Nicolle, Jacques. *Louis Pasteur: The Story of His Major Discoveries*. New York: Basic Books, 1961.

Parish, Henry James. *Victory with Vaccines: The Story of Immunization*. Edinburgh, London: E. & S. Livingstone, 1968.

Rains, A. J. Harding. *Edward Jenner and Vaccination*. London: Priory Press, 1974.

Razzell, P. E. *The Conquest of Smallpox: The Impact of Inoculation on Smallpox Mortality in Eighteenth Century Britain*. Firle: Caliban Books, 1977.

Saunders, Paul. *Edward Jenner, the Cheltenham Years, 1795–1823: Being a Chronicle of the Vaccination Campaign*. Hanover, NH: University Press of New England, 1982.

Smith, Jane S. *Patenting the Sun: Polio and the Salk Vaccine*. New York: William Morrow, 1990.

Smith, Jane S. *Patenting the Sun: Polio and the Salk Vaccine*. New York: Anchor/Doubleday, 1991.

Vallery-Radot, René. *The Life of Pasteur*. New York: Dover Publications, 1960.

THE EXPERTS' FORUM

Mothering has brought together a group of five healthcare practitioners interested in and knowledgeable about vaccinations. They represent different health and vaccine philosophies and were each asked to answer the same questions regarding vaccinations. The questions were developed by our editor in conjunction with parents and the participants in the forum.

What this forum represents is hours of nearly free medical consultation on vaccinations. The participating doctors gave a great deal to this effort, sending additional material, laboring over answers, and responding to one another in the editing process. Each has made a major and significant contribution.

The Experts' Forum also includes several short articles written by the participants, as well as charts. These charts, which compare risks and symptoms of diseases with risks and effectiveness of vaccines, were prepared by our editor with information sent or referred to by the participants.

The participants in the Experts' Forum include Miranda Castro, Jay Gordon, Anne Montgomery, Richard Moskowitz, and Barbara Watson.

Miranda Castro, FSHom, is a professional homeopath and a fellow of the Society of Homeopaths in the United Kingdom. She is the author of *The Complete Homeopathy Handbook*, *Homeopathy for Pregnancy, Birth and Your Baby's First Year*, and *Homeopathic Solutions for Emotional and Physical Stress*. She is currently on the faculty of Bastyr University in Seattle, Washington.

Jay Gordon, MD, is board certified in pediatrics and is an instructor with the UCLA School of Medicine and the Cedars-Sinai Medical Center, on the faculty of the Lactation Institute, and a member of the Medical Advisory Board of La Leche League International. He is the author of *Good Food Today* and *Great Kids Tomorrow*, and practices family medicine in Santa Monica, California.

Anne Montgomery, MD, is board certified in family practice and is assistant editor of the *Journal of Human Lactation*. She is a clinical assistant professor in the Department of Family Practice, University of Washington Medical School, and a faculty physician with St. Peter Hospital Family Residency Program, Olympia, Washington.

Richard Moskowitz, MD, is the author of *Homeopathic Medicines for Pregnancy and Childbirth* and is a member of the teaching faculty of the National Center for Homeopathy, the International Foundation for Homeopathy, and the College of Homeopathy. He practices general and family medicine with an emphasis on classical homeopathy, patient education, and advocacy. He has published articles, essays, and other works on homeopathy, vaccinations, and related topics.

Barbara Watson, MD, is a medical vaccination specialist currently associated with the Vaccine Development Center at the Children's Hospital of Philadelphia, the University of Pennsylvania School of Medicine, and the Philadelphia Department of Public Health. She has published numerous papers and abstracts on vaccinations and related topics.

1. HOW DOES NATURAL IMMUNITY WORK?

MONTGOMERY: There are several components to the body's defense against infection. The ability to avoid becoming ill with a disease to which one is exposed depends on the general health of the individual, the health of the immune system as a whole, and the presence of specific immunity to that particular disease. It also depends on the infectivity (chance of developing infection after exposure) and virulence (likelihood of virus to cause clinically apparent illness) of the virus or bacterium that causes the disease. Some bacteria or viruses cause infection only in people with immune system dysfunction; others cause disease in almost anyone who is exposed to them. In many cases, people with healthy immune systems have mild illnesses, while people with poor immune systems, or decreased disease-specific immunity, have severe illnesses. Age also plays a role: measles and chickenpox are generally mild diseases in young children but can be severe and even fatal in a relatively large percentage of adults; *Hemophilus influenzae* type b and pertussis can cause severe disease in young infants but usually cause relatively mild disease in healthy older children and adults.

The immune system is quite complex and includes many different disease-fighting components. Some white blood cells (neutrophils, T-lymphocytes, macrophages) fight viruses or bacteria directly; other (B-lymphocytes) make antibodies which are specific proteins that attach to the virus or bacteria and make it more obvious to the disease-fighting cells. These B-lymphocytes develop specific "immunologic memory," continuing to make a low level of antibody even after the disease has run its course. Natural disease-specific immunity, acquired after exposure to and recovery from a natural infection, consists of both antibody-mediated and cell-mediated immunity; the whole immune system works together. When the individual is reexposed to the same disease, the specific antibody level rises rapidly, and the individual does not redevelop symptoms of the disease. Viruses such as measles and chickenpox generally produce lifelong immunity after a single episode of disease. Other viruses, such as influenza, change rapidly, so people can be reinfected every year as a new strain of influenza comes along.

Sometimes active natural immunity can develop even without clinical symptoms of disease. For example, about 70 percent of adults who say they have not had chickenpox do have antibodies to varicella, the chickenpox virus. However, the immune system is immature in young children under two years of age or so; sometimes children who have a very mild case of disease such as chickenpox when they are very young do not develop lifetime immunity to that disease. Many of the symptoms of disease (fever, for example) are really manifestations of the body's reaction to the infectious agent and thus tend to be more severe when the immune system is more "mature," somewhat ironically leading to more severe illness in older children and adults. This also leads to a greater immune response and "better immunity" in these people with more mature immune systems. In general, people at greatest risk for serious complications of infectious disease are the very young (premies and young infants), the very old, and the immunocompromised.

In addition to active natural immunity developed in reaction to exposures, infants have natural passive immunity. Antibodies are passed from the mother to the infant during the last few months of pregnancy, so the full-term newborn has some immunity to all diseases to which its mother has the long-term blood-borne antibody (IgG). This immunity provides the greatest protection just after birth and gradually declines over about a year. It also provides more protection against some diseases (e.g., measles, rubella, tetanus) than others (e.g., polio, pertussis).

Some passive immunity continues through breastfeeding, particularly antibodies (IgA class) and immune cells that act locally in the respiratory and gastrointestinal tracts. Breastfed babies/children in general have healthier immune systems and so may have less severe illnesses. However, breastfeeding does not provide the same specific disease-related immunity that is acquired before birth, through active exposure to disease or through immunization, because specific immune factors are not absorbed intact from the gastrointestinal tract. Breastfed children generally have a stronger response to immunization and develop higher levels of immunity after receiving vaccinations than do formula-fed children.

2. WHAT ARE VACCINES? HOW DOES VACCINE IMMUNITY WORK?

GORDON: Vaccines are fragments of bacterial or viral material that fool the immune system into thinking that there is an ongoing infection. Vaccines can be "killed"—that is, totally inactivated—or "live," wherein the organism has been damaged so that it cannot cause infection but is still not completely dead. Vaccines also contain preservatives and other chemicals.

The immune system seems to respond with the same type of antibody production that occurs with an actual infection, but there may not be the same amount or type of antibody produced. The immunity may not last as long as natural immunity.

MONTGOMERY: The concept of introducing an alternative substance in order to induce active immunity against a disease developed from the observation that persons who had cowpox did not develop smallpox. In fact, the word *vaccine* comes from *vacca*, Latin for "cow." In the severe smallpox epidemics of the 15th and 16th centuries, milkmaids who had cowpox, a much milder illness, did not develop smallpox, a severe disease that caused many deaths. Early vaccines were developed using the concept of introducing a milder form of the bacteria or virus in order to induce immunity without causing severe disease.

Subsequently, vaccines have also been developed that use inactivated (or "killed") organisms and that use only components of organisms. These vaccines work because antibodies are directed at components of the virus or bacteria called "antigens," most commonly protein or complex sugar components of the outer membrane or wall of the organism. The common childhood vaccines we use today include all of these types of vaccines.

Live-attenuated vaccines are made in laboratories from viruses and bacteria that have been specially weakened so that they lead to immunity but not to illness. They create immunity by "infecting" the individual and growing and reproducing within the body, just like native bacteria and viruses do. They induce immunity that is essentially the same as natural disease-specific immunity. This infection is usually not symptomatic but can result in illness in some cases, particularly in people with depressed immune systems. The individual develops long-lasting immunity that includes both antibody- and cell-mediated immunity. Generally, only one shot is needed in the initial series, although, as with measles, we have discovered that the immunity is not necessarily as long-lasting as naturally acquired immunity. Previously present antibodies can interfere with the action of live-attenuated vaccines, so most of these are given after the prenatally acquired antibody has cleared (after the first birthday). Attenuated live virus vaccines available now include measles, mumps, rubella, polio (OPV), yellow fever, vaccinia, and varicella. Live-attenuated bacterial vaccines include BCG (tuberculosis) and typhoid (a recombinant vaccine).

Inactivated vaccines may use the whole killed organism or a portion of the organism. Because they are not living organisms, they cannot cause disease. However, they do not lead to as strong an immune response. Whole-virus vaccines in general cause more side effects than do more purified component vaccines. Inactivated vaccines always require multiple doses, usually three to five. Most of these vaccines also need boosters because immunity falls over time. They are not, however, affected by circulating antibodies and so can be effective given in infancy. Whole-cell inactivated vaccines include influenza, polio (IPV), rabies, and hepatitis A viruses, pertussis, typhoid, cholera, and plague bacteria. Subunit vaccines (made from pieces of the microorganisms) include the first hepatitis B vaccine, influenza, and the acellular pertussis vaccine. The newer hepatitis B vaccine is a synthetic component rather than a piece of native virus. Diphtheria and tetanus vaccines are toxoids, a protein-only component.

Polysaccharide vaccines are a subtype of inactivated vaccine. The body tends to respond more strongly to protein components than to the complex sugar molecules called polysaccharides that make up the outer wall of some bacteria. Polysaccharide vaccines such as those for pneumococcus and meningococcus do not work in children under age two and do not have a booster effect. The *Hemophilus influenzae* type b vaccine is a polysaccharide that has been attached (conjugated) to a protein, which seems to have eliminated these problems.

There are a number of new vaccine strategies being developed as a result of genetic engineering, with the goal of inducing the most effective immunity with the least side effects. The newer hepatitis B vaccine was the first licensed recombinant vaccine. Some live vaccines are being modified so they will engender the best "natural" immunity without the risk of causing disease.

WATSON: The term *vaccine* is derived from *Vaccinia* ("smallpox"), which was the first scientific use of disease prevention, although attempts to immunize are almost as old as attempts to eradicate disease. The Chinese treated smallpox with inoculation as early as the sixth century. A report of a Buddhist nun using the scabs from smallpox lesions and blowing them into nostrils is described in A.D. 1022. A vaccine is the use of an antigen that has been altered, such that it will not cause disease but will produce the appropriate immune response to protect the body from that agent when it meets it in the environment.

How does vaccine immunity work? It depends on the type of vaccine, but the basic immune recognition of the antigen (vaccine), or any disease-causing agent for that matter, and the production of antibodies with or without the cell-mediated immune response component is the key. For example, scientists discovered that persons with antibodies to PRP (polyribotol phosphate), a sugar from the outer membrane of the organism *Hemophilus influenzae* type b, which causes meningitis, were protected from the disease. They also found that children under five lacked antibodies, and that most of the cases of Hib meningitis occur in children under five. Thus, a vaccine using purified PRP was made. However, infants have an immature immune system that needs the help of protein antigens, such as tetanus toxoid, to be able to recognize the sugar or PRP.

The dose of vaccine administered has to be sufficient to stimulate the immune response, not overwhelm it. Usually with pure protein vaccines and killed organisms or toxoids, several doses are required. Thus, the need for clinical trials to establish just how many doses are required to achieve a protective antibody level during a person's period of greatest risk of contracting the disease. Live-attenuated vaccines usually only need to be given once, as the agent multiplies in the vaccinee; thus the number of immune cells recruited during the replication process is greater than when a killed agent is used. Also, the immune response can be augmented by adding adjuvants, such as alum, which stimulate a greater recruitment of immune cells to the site of the vaccine.

MOSKOWITZ: Vaccines are either inactivated preparations, toxins, or extracts from disease-causing microbes (e.g., pertussis and Hib vaccines, diphtheria and tetanus toxoids), or live bacteria or viruses that have been specifically attenuated to the point that they are much less likely to provoke acute disease.

Unlike the acute or wild-type infections they are designed to prevent, vaccines that are introduced directly into the blood, bypassing the normal portal of entry, produce no massive immune system outpouring, and are intended to elicit a measurable titers of specific antibodies for long periods of time. Such a feat could only be accomplished if vaccines remained antigenically active in the antibody-producing cells of the host more or less indefinitely, with no obvious means of getting rid of them.

I am not yet certain about how this happens, but my clinical experience confirms what my knowledge of microbiology suggests— that, insofar as they work at all, vaccines work by rendering the host less likely to respond acutely, not only to the virus or bacterium in question but nonspecifically to other foreign and infectious agents, as well.

In other words, people vaccinated against measles, say, are less likely to come down with the typical acute case of measles because they already have chronic measles, so to speak, and have also been reprogrammed to respond chronically to other such threats in the future.

3. IS THERE A COST TO THE IMMUNE SYSTEM FOR THE IMMUNITY FROM VACCINATION? DOES THE IMMUNE SYSTEM HAVE A FINITE CAPACITY?

CASTRO: The crux of this issue is not that vaccination isn't sometimes effective but that it may be so at a cost to health. Natural exposure to bacteria and viruses causes a generalized inflammatory response that protects the major organs and tissues from those foreign particles. When the vaccine is absorbed into the bloodstream, it bypasses the body's normal lines of defense and has direct access to the major organs and tissues, eliciting a particular type of antibody response that the body normally uses only as a last resort. While the individual may have some resistance to a particular disease, the body's ability to react against other infections is reduced, i.e., the immune system acts as if it is overloaded, and this may lead to a general lowering of resistance.

The immune system can be enhanced and strengthened, particularly through good nutrition (including having been breastfed as a baby), adequate rest and sleep, exercise, the avoidance of unnecessary drugs and medications, satisfying relationships, and so forth. Conversely, it can be stressed and weakened through such things as poor nutrition, emotional stress, a lack of exercise, and unnecessary drugs and medications. While the immune system is remarkably resilient and appears to have almost limitless powers of recovery, one that is stressed to its own limit can and will break down.

GORDON: From a conventional medical point of view, there seems to be little or no cost to the immune system from vaccination. A more broadminded approach would suggest that there has to be some cost when the immune system is "distracted" and asked to produce diphtheria antibodies in the middle of the winter cold season, when it might be otherwise fully engaged dealing with the more common "bug *du jour.*" The immune system probably does not have a finite capacity in children, but the theories that say it does cannot be disproved and therefore must be considered as possible.

MONTGOMERY: I believe the answer to this question is no. Most of the studies of vaccination indicate that virtually any combination of vaccines can be given together and still be effective, and that mild illness is not a contraindication to vaccination. There are millions of T cells, B cells, and so forth in the body. It's hard to imagine enough diseases to overwhelm all of them. Vaccines particularly are not likely to "cost" the immune system very much since we only routinely vaccinate against about ten diseases in children. Kids get exposed to four to six different strains of cold virus plus a few gastroenterologic viruses and several bacteria each year. They must respond to each one with a new immune response. In other words, the proportion of the work the immune system does that is directed at vaccines is pretty minimal.

Most of us as parents have observed that our children seem to get sick shortly after receiving their immunizations, or that they seem to get one cold after another, and we wonder if the immune system is getting overwhelmed and becoming unable to fight off the next thing that comes along. Kids get sick because other kids get sick and share their germs. Unless there is a significant problem with the immune system, vaccines are not likely to have any major effect on the body's ability to deal with other diseases. For immunocompromised kids, for those with chronic diseases, and for those who are recovering from a particularly serious illness, some modification of the immunization schedule may be in order.

WATSON: Is there a cost to the immune system for the immunity from vaccination? No, the cost is the same as that of living in an environment that has a number of organisms with which we share the planet.

Does the immune system have a finite capacity? This question appears to come from the concern that immunization will use up some of the immune system's "limited capacity." The short answer to this question for *healthy* individuals is no. Our strongest immune responses come between the ages of five and 25—if we are well-nourished, well-rested, not under excess mental or emotional stress or deprivation, and not concurrently infected with an organism, such as the EBV or CMV viruses, which impair the immune system, or a disease process, or medications (including some herbal remedies) that impair the immune system. Cells age, and as we grow older, the immune system is less able to perform. At the same time, when the immune system is immature it is less able to process some antigens.

MOSKOWITZ: Yes. The principal cost is the inherently counterfeit nature of vaccine-mediated "immunity." Natural immunity acquired by recovery from acute illness such as measles is ordinarily absolute and lifelong, such that, no matter how many epidemics the individual may be exposed to in the future, the risk of reinfection is practically zero.

Indeed, I would argue that the ability to mount and recover from acute infection, to respond acutely and vigorously to foreign microbial agents, is the chief stimulus for the maturation of a healthy immune system, representing a net gain for the health not only of the individual but ultimately of the species as well.

Artificial or vaccine-related "immunity," on the other hand, is at best the substitution of chronic illness for acute illness, which is rather like taking out a mortgage at a very high rate of interest amortized over the patient's lifetime—hardly a good trade-off in my view. Mandatory vaccination is really a kind of genetic engineering, producing recombinant forms of bacterial and viral DNA within the antibody-producing cells of the blood, with potentially ominous consequences for the future of the race.

It has taken many centuries of experience with the measles virus to convert it from a major killer into a routine disease of childhood, such that, when I was first exposed to it at the age of six, nonspecific mechanisms were already in place to expedite my recovery. Today, the milk of vaccinated mothers no longer contains measles antibodies, and tiny infants too young to be vaccinated are once more coming down with it, as are adolescents and young adults of reproductive age, the very groups who most need to be protected.

By allowing the production of specific antibodies, the end result of immunity, to stand for the whole process that made it possible, vaccination confers a partial lowering of susceptibility to acute infection along with an increased vulnerability to chronic diseases, both in childhood and in later life. As more and more vaccines are added to the pile, as if they were beneficial and risk-free without qualification or limit, I fear that we are like the sorcerer's apprentice, unknowingly precipitating an evolutionary crisis of major proportions.

4. ARE VACCINES EFFECTIVE? WHAT PROOF DO WE HAVE OF THIS?

GORDON: Vaccines are very effective. In spite of the graphs that suggest a decline in certain illnesses before vaccines were used, these illnesses were greatly lessened or, in a few cases, eliminated by the vaccines against them.

In my practice, I have a large number of unvaccinated or partially vaccinated children. When pertussis comes to town, as it does every few years, the preponderance of cases is in the unvaccinated population.

Literally thousands of studies have been done showing the efficacy of vaccines. The FDA and similar agencies require these studies prior to approving a new vaccine.

MONTGOMERY: None of our vaccines provides lifelong immunity to everyone who receives it, but all of the currently recommended vaccines have been shown to induce immunity in a large percentage of recipients and to reduce the incidence of disease.

Vaccine efficacy can be studied in several ways. Efficacy from a population standpoint looks at the overall incidence of disease as compared to the vaccination rate. For example, nearly 99 percent of people vaccinated against measles have antibodies; about 95 percent of them do not develop disease upon exposure. The incidence of disease has fallen with the increasing vaccination rate, and in the cases of measles, mumps, rubella, and so forth, risen again when the vaccination rate in the population has decreased.

I would like to point out a pitfall in looking at absolute numbers of cases rather than disease rates, as is sometimes done to challenge claims of vaccine efficacy. In a highly vaccinated population, it is likely that a large proportion of the cases of a disease will occur in vaccinated individuals. This does not mean that the vaccine is ineffective. For example, assume that out of 1,000 kids, 980 are vaccinated against measles and 20 aren't. Statistically, 39 of the vaccinated children will become infected during an outbreak, as will 18 unvaccinated children. Hence, one could conclude that more measles occurred in vaccinated than in unvaccinated children, but it is more accurate to say that 90 percent of unvaccinated children got measles, and only 4 percent of vaccinated kids got measles. The vaccine was quite effective but not perfect.

WATSON: Yes, vaccines are effective. With the exception of safe water, nothing—not even antibiotics—has had such an effect on disease reduction and population growth.

5. IS IT TRUE THAT THE INCIDENCE OF SOME DISEASES DECLINED BEFORE VACCINATIONS FOR THEM WERE INTRODUCED? IS THE OVERALL DECLINE IN DISEASE RELATED TO IMPROVED HEALTH AND SANITATION OR TO VACCINATIONS, OR BOTH?

MONTGOMERY: Public health measures have certainly contributed to the decline in many diseases and the virtual elimination of pandemics of diseases such as were seen with the plague in Europe and even with influenza in this century. However, all vaccine-preventable diseases have declined since the vaccine was introduced, some quite dramatically. If one were to plot the incidence of vaccine-preventable diseases such as diphtheria, pertussis, measles, and polio (wild), the trend over the last 40 to 60 years is up and down with an overall gradual downward trend until the vaccine was introduced, followed by a precipitous decline to 97 to 100 percent lower levels. More recently, the incidence of Hib meningitis, a life-threatening disease of young infants, has declined to almost zero in many areas since the introduction of the vaccine in the 1980s.

MOSKOWITZ: Unquestionably, the measles vaccine has been effective in reducing the incidence of acute measles in the US from over 400,000 cases annually in the prevaccine era to less than 10,000 from the late 1960s until today. Similar results have been observed with regard to polio, mumps, and rubella. The data for Hib, an organism that is regularly present in healthy children, as well, and for hepatitis B, which is a disease of IV drug users, their sexual partners, and medical and surgical patients receiving contaminated blood via transfusion, will not be unequivocally known for some time, if ever.

6. IF DISEASES HAVE A LIFE CYCLE, AND MOST OF THE ONES WE VACCINATE AGAINST ARE ON THE DECLINE, THEN WHAT IS THE FEAR OF NOT VACCINATING? IS IT COMMON FOR DISEASES ON THE DECLINE TO HAVE A SIGNIFICANT RESURGENCE?

GORDON: It is common for diseases to run in cycles and epidemics. A disease that appears to be on the way out can have a strong resurgence for a variety of reasons, not the least of which may be declining immunization rates as people worry less: Witness the small but significant measles epidemics in the past five years and the polio outbreaks in Amsterdam, Israel, and elsewhere in the past five to ten years. Vaccinations possibly carry a risk not well acknowledged by the conventional medical community, but stopping certain vaccines will undoubtedly lead to an increase in these illnesses.

MONTGOMERY: Most of the diseases we immunize for have been around for a very long time (centuries or longer) and are only finally on their way out because of the immunizations. Their overall incidence was declining, but they weren't gone. It is not common to have pandemics of any of them anymore, but it is pretty common to still have epidemics—of measles, for example. Pertussis has also been on the rise again in the past few years, probably due to the increasing number of children not vaccinated against pertussis and also (as with measles) to the decreased boosters past age seven. Unless a disease is completely eliminated, it certainly can have a resurgence.

There has been much discussion about whether to destroy the smallpox virus that is being held in secure labs in Atlanta and Moscow. Smallpox has been eliminated from the world, and there is concern that the virus could be used as a biological weapon. However, there is also concern that smallpox could spontaneously recur as a mutation, from the cowpox virus for example, and without the virus in the lab, we wouldn't be able to rapidly redevelop vaccine. The HIV epidemic has shown how a disease can spread in a susceptible population, even in the late 20th century, and also raises concern because of the large number of people now infected with HIV who may be susceptible to other diseases.

Outbreaks of pertussis in Japan and Great Britain and polio in Finland preclude complacency even about diseases that are now uncommon in the US.

Is it likely that not vaccinating one child will lead to the resurgence of a disease? Of course not. But it is likely that if large numbers of children go unvaccinated, there will be sufficient reservoirs of disease to lead to some local outbreaks and possibly to epidemics. Global travel also increases the risk of outbreaks when unvaccinated people travel to endemic areas, or people from endemic areas travel to areas in which the vaccination rate is low. Pandemics are unlikely since we have much better public health measures now and also could respond to an outbreak with a targeted vaccination program, which would prevent further spread.

WATSON: Diseases do not die out on their own. As long as there is a *susceptible* "host" for the agent and ongoing *transmission*, the disease can continue to afflict persons on the earth. The diseases against which we vaccinate are on the decline because we have cut down on the number of susceptible hosts or improved immunity such that transmission cannot continue.

However, we must never forget that the US is not isolated from the rest of the world. Until all other countries in the world reach the same high levels of immunity to disease, importation of an agent/disease, such as measles or the Ebola virus, poses a danger to anyone who is not immune. In Philadelphia in 1989, a case of measles imported from Spain by an unimmunized traveler started an epidemic that sickened 1,550 children and killed nine; 31 percent of the cases occurred in children who should have received their vaccines, i.e., children older than 16 months. In New York there were 3,000 cases of measles and 24 deaths in 1990 and 1991. There are many examples of resurgence of disease in areas where immunization takes a backseat to war or, as in Russia, political unrest. If an agent's *only* host is the human, then disease eradication is feasible; the example we have is smallpox. The political will to rid the world of smallpox back in the 1960s and 1970s was equal to the efforts placed to put a man on the moon! Eradication of disease and maintenance of surveillance until the disease is eradicated worldwide require global commitment.

MOSKOWITZ: Infectious diseases become epidemic in certain waves or rhythmic cycles, vaccine or no vaccine. Diphtheria, for example, has been all but eliminated in Europe, but even by present criteria, the level of immunity in vaccinated adults is so low that authorities are now predicting it will reappear. Likewise, the level of apparent immunity from specific antibodies to rubella is about the same in vaccinated kids today as it was in the prevaccine era.

7. HOW DO VACCINATED AND NONVACCINATED CHILDREN COMPARE REGARDING INCIDENCE AND SEVERITY OF DISEASE?

GORDON: It has been my personal experience that nonvaccinated children get sick less often and that some children get their first illness right after the first vaccine. I'm not aware of any studies that back up my anecdotal data. This is also a skewed sample group because these families may be breastfeeding longer, may smoke a lot less, may eat better, may be more health-conscious, and so forth. In other words, this is *not* a scientific study on my part, eliminating the effect of other variables.

MONTGOMERY: An individual's manifestation of infection varies with many factors. Most of the vaccines we have are more than 90 percent effective, meaning 2 to 15 percent of vaccinated kids will get sick during an outbreak. This compares with probably 70 to 95 percent of unvaccinated kids getting sick when exposed, depending on the disease. However, most of our vaccine-preventable diseases are no longer very common, so most nonvaccinated kids won't be exposed anyway and therefore won't get sick.

A vaccinated kid with immunity will not get sick when exposed. Vaccinated kids who did not develop immunity will get sick when exposed in the same proportion to unvaccinated kids. However, depending on the disease, sometimes kids who did not show significant antibody response to the vaccine will have less severe illness. This is particularly true for those who initially responded but later lost their immunity; they usually maintain some immunologic memory and thus fight off the infection more efficiently. Kids who have been partially immunized but have not completed the whole vaccination series have a higher rate of disease than fully vaccinated kids, lower than unvaccinated kids. When they do contract a disease for which they have partial immunity, they generally have less severe illness.

MOSKOWITZ: On the whole, with many of the acute diseases in question, vaccinated kids are somewhat less likely to get them when exposed than their unvaccinated couterparts. Overall, this is probably true of measles, mumps, rubella, polio, pertussis, and tetanus. On the other hand, when these diseases do break out, significant numbers of vaccinated kids also get them, and when the vaccination rate approaches 100 percent, as in the measles epidemics of the 1980s, the vast majority of the cases are vaccinated.

8. WHY DO SCHOOLS KEEP NONVACCINATED CHILDREN AT HOME WHEN THERE'S AN OUTBREAK OF DISEASE? ARE NONVACCINATED CHILDREN A RISK TO VACCINATED CHILDREN? UNDER WHAT CIRCUMSTANCES SHOULD WE KEEP OUR CHILDREN AWAY FROM ONE ANOTHER? ARE CHILDREN WHO HAVE RECENTLY BEEN VACCINATED WITH LIVE POLIO A RISK TO OTHERS?

GORDON: Schools keep nonvaccinated children home during an outbreak of disease to slow or stop the outbreak. This is a correct intervention as far as I'm concerned, protecting both the unvaccinated children and their classmates from a more widespread epidemic. But children who have recently received the polio vaccine pose no real threat to other children. They may cause polio in an immunocompromised person, such as someone with AIDS or undergoing cancer chemotherapy. These children will probably accidentally vaccinate their unvaccinated classmates as they shed the vaccine in their saliva and stool for weeks or months after having taken the oral polio vaccine. We probably do not need to keep kids away from other kids who have received the vaccines except in the above-mentioned instances. During a pertussis outbreak, I would definitely take extra care with my unvaccinated child.

MONTGOMERY: Nonvaccinated kids are kept at home during an outbreak primarily to keep them from getting sick. A secondary consideration is that nonvaccinated kids serve as a reservoir of disease since all diseases have an incubation period and are infectious before the kid becomes sick. The danger to vaccinated kids is only to that small percentage of them who were vaccinated but did not develop immunity. In general, during outbreaks, the public health goal is to limit the total number of people who get sick, so keeping people who could catch the disease away from people who have the disease until the last case has run its course is the usual preference. Of course, this prevents nonvaccinated kids from developing natural disease-specific immunity during an outbreak; if that's what the parents hoped for when they chose not to vaccinate, then the "quarantine" is not what they want. Again, it's important to remember that some of these diseases, notably measles, cause mild disease in young children but cause severe disease in older children and adults. Reservoirs of disease can lead to outbreaks that spread to adults who are not immune, including pregnant women and high-risk groups such as HIV-infected persons.

WATSON: Schools keep nonvaccinated children at home because they are not immune and will get the disease and also serve as new hosts to continue the transmission of the outbreak. Nonvaccinated kids are not a risk to appropriately vaccinated kids; however, they serve as a potential reservoir for disease outbreaks.

Live-attenuated polio vaccine (OPV) is shed from 24 hours to six weeks after the first dose. Once an individual has antibody, the duration of shedding decreases significantly. Unvaccinated individuals (persons who have never had a polio shot or who are immunocompromised such that they have low antibodies to OPV) are at risk if they have close contact with a child shedding OPV. Hence, the current debate on inactivated polio vaccine versus OPV.

As a general rule of "infection control," healthy *nonimmune* individuals should stay away from anyone with a contagious disease. For example, if you have a newborn, and an older sibling has a cough that may be pertussis, RSV, influenza, or TB, it is ideal that the nonimmune infant (one who has not been immunized) be separated from the contagious older sibling.

MOSKOWITZ: Good question. If vaccines conferred a genuine immunity, then the unvaccinated kids would be a threat only to themselves, and it would be totally unnecessary to keep them home from school when an epidemic of something breaks out. Conversely, the paranoia about unvaccinated kids is itself a measure of the ineffectiveness of the vaccines, even by their own test.

Indeed, in the case of the oral polio at least, the shoe is on the other foot, and the unvaccinated kids are at some very small risk of acquiring the virus from their newly vaccinated friends, as are the vaccinated children's parents and siblings, for that matter. Certainly, as a practical matter, it makes good common sense to keep sick kids home from school but not to penalize unvaccinated kids for exercising their legal rights in the absence of any public health emergency.

9. VACCINES ARE RECOMMENDED FOR YOUNGER AND YOUNGER INFANTS. ARE EARLY VACCINES APPROPRIATE FOR ALL INFANTS? IS DELAYING SOME OR ALL VACCINES A RESPONSIBLE OPTION?

CASTRO: In my opinion this needs challenging. It is one aspect of vaccination that concerns me. Vaccines are by definition toxic, and those injected into an infant's bloodstream represent a serious assault on an immune system that is still in the early stages of its development.

They should be delayed for as long as possible in order to give an infant's immune system a chance to mature. In the UK, doctors have been advised to vaccinate earlier in order to ensure a higher rate of patient compliance—some are recommending the first DPT at four weeks old. Research is urgently needed (and some is under way in the UK) to demonstrate that this practice is detrimental to the general health of the infant.

I think all vaccinations should be delayed until at least six months, in order to give the infant's immune system a chance to form itself (and be judged as healthy) before being exposed to vaccine stresses.

GORDON: I believe we may be vaccinating our babies too early, but part of the rationale for doing this is: "Let's stick 'em while we got 'em." That is, some families drop out of routine health care for a variety of reasons—economic, social, and others. If we vaccinate early, we have the greatest chance of retaining "herd immunity." Delaying some or all vaccines may be a very responsible option.

I think that some families stop vaccinating—or don't vaccinate at all—because they feel pressured to give a shot or two or three to a newborn or to a six-week-old infant. I counsel the families in my practice to read about immunizations, put a lot of thought into the issue, ask lots of questions, and vaccinate when they are more comfortable with the whole idea.

MONTGOMERY: I'd like to start this discussion with some reflection on vaccination policies. As parents, we need to make decisions about our children's health as individuals. The people who decide vaccine recommendations are also concerned with the health of individual children, but their job is to make public health policy. Public health policy tries to get the most good for the society at the least cost to the society as a whole. Parents need to keep this in mind as they make decisions. Most of us want to be good citizens and to participate in things that benefit society as a whole, but it is true that the application of public health policy to individual people doesn't always work.

In order to eliminate disease in a society through vaccination, the majority, if not all, of the people must be vaccinated. The only time we see people in the healthcare system often enough to complete the primary series of vaccination is in the first years of life. From a public health standpoint, it makes absolutely the most sense to give as many vaccines as we can as early as we can, and as many at the same time as we can. This provides the best chance to immunize the greatest portion of the population. Targeting a vaccination program solely toward people at high risk for contracting hepatitis B failed to have much impact on the prevalence of the disease; the change to a universal recommendation for infant vaccination is starting to make a difference. We won't know for many years how many cases of liver cancer we have prevented, but it will be a substantial number. In addition, many vaccines cost less to administer to younger children because of smaller doses or fewer shots required.

Some of the vaccine-preventable diseases, notably Hib and pertussis, clearly cause severe disease in young infants. Other vaccine-preventable diseases, such as hepatitis B, are common in some subpopulations of children (notably Asian immigrant families) and uncommon in children in other groups. Hepatitis B, however, becomes a significant threat for some sexually active adolescents and adults in all populations. Other diseases, such as rubella, are very mild, except that they are devastating to fetuses, so we vaccinate in order to keep pregnant women from contracting the disease. The new recommendations about varicella take into consideration the huge dollar cost of parental time lost from work (a topic for philosophical discussion in itself).

For healthy breastfed babies cared for at home, I do not have much quarrel with parents who wish to delay other immunizations, although I do encourage full vaccination on a schedule with which the parents are comfortable. For most babies, I think it is easiest to just follow the vaccination schedule at the time of their well-baby visits, but I don't think it is irresponsible to thoughtfully delay some of the immunizations, particularly for diseases that have become pretty uncommon. (I do find it irresponsible to decide to vaccinate and then neglect to follow through with timely vaccination.) Premature infants are a special case, since they don't get the full complement of maternal antibodies before birth and may be more likely to suffer significant consequences from infection with some of these diseases; probably premies should be immunized on schedule. I do feel that children who will be in daycare should be fully immunized, however, for their own individual protection as well as for public health reasons.

WATSON: Vaccines are recommended for younger and younger infants. Our tremendous gain in knowledge about the immune system over the last 15 years has led to recommendations for earlier immunization. Recommendations for the timing of immunizations balance the age at which the immune system will respond to the vaccine with the child's risk from the disease. For example, a newborn is at great risk for life-threatening complications should he or she contract measles, but the maternal antibodies passed on through breast-feeding and the infant's immaturity make the vaccine ineffective at this age. By 12 months of age, the risk from the disease is still great, maternal antibodies have faded (even in breastfed babies), and the immune system is receptive to the vaccine, and so the measles vaccine is now recommended at this time. Prior to the 1980s, the recommended age was 15 months, but it has been reduced to 12 months because most young mothers now (born in the 1960s) were immunized with MMR, and their level of immunity is lower.

In the rest of the world, where access to health care is problematic, and the only time all infants come into contact with a healthcare worker is at birth, the ideal would be to devise a vaccine that could be given at birth orally, and would time-release each antigen appropriately.

10. ARE SOME VACCINES RISKIER THAN OTHERS?

CASTRO: Yes (tetanus appears to be the most benign), but we cannot predict the individual's reaction to vaccination. Unfortunately, trying to weigh the risk factors against the benefits of vaccination is like playing Russian roulette because many outcomes are simply not predictable.

GORDON: The pertussis vaccine is the riskiest of the common vaccines. Unfortunately, whooping cough is the most common illness against which we vaccinate our children. The disease itself, while rarely fatal, is a long, scary illness that can put a child in the hospital, cause seizures, and has a 1/200 mortality rate in children in the first two months of life.

WATSON: The word *risky* is inaccurate and implies unknown side effects, but the DTP is more *reactive* (causes more fever, fretfulness, drowsiness, or soreness in the leg at injection site) than DT, APDT, MMR, Hib, HepB, varicella, or yellow fever. In travel vaccines, earlier versions of typhoid, cholera, rabies, and Japanese encephalitis vaccines were more reactive than versions available today. This is another reason for promoting research on vaccine development.

MOSKOWITZ: Yes. Not only must each vaccine be considered separately, but the risk of the corresponding disease is also somewhat different in each case. Thus, tetanus toxoid might be worth giving to a healthy three year old who lives and plays around horses, whereas giving hepatitis B to all newborns because of our inability to target the drug users is criminal.

The MMR is a good example of a vaccine with considerable risk and virtually no benefit, directed against diseases that our natural herd immunity had already dealt with effectively and adding significantly to our general chronic disease burden. The oral polio is somewhat risky because of contamination with other monkey viruses during the attenuation process.

The Hib and pneumococcus vaccines are the first of a long line of newer vaccines directed against organisms commonly harbored in healthy children that are occasionally associated with serious disease. Vaccines against hemolytic *Streptococci* are already in the pipeline. Where will it end? Why not *E. coli* and the intestinal bacteria, which do many good things for us but also can be pathogenic at times? What about *Staphylococci*, yeast, and other inhabitants of the skin and vagina that occasionally make trouble?

The truth is that biotech firms are busy cranking out new genetically engineered vaccines against many different organisms for no other reason than their technical capacity to make them. Merck has been sitting on the chickenpox vaccine for 25 years, until the current provaccine hysteria provided the rationale for marketing it.

11. WHEN VACCINE REACTIONS DO OCCUR, IS IT THE VACCINE TOXIN ITSELF, THE CULTURING MEDIUM ON WHICH THE VACCINE IS GROWN, ADDITIVES AND PRESERVATIVES, OR THE SENSITIVITY OF THE PERSON RECEIVING THE VACCINE THAT ACCOUNTS FOR THE REACTION?

CASTRO: Any or all of the above are capable of producing reactions. One double-blind trial using the vaccines in one group and the medium in a control group showed serious side effects in both groups. Each substance used in the manufacture of vaccines is potentially toxic. As with other medications, a list of ingredients would help parents in their decision making.

MONTGOMERY: Yes, all of these contribute. People can react to the vaccine. The culturing medium (usually egg) and additive such as neomycin can cause allergic reactions in susceptible individuals. The preservative thimerosal is present in several vaccines and can cause a local hypersensitivity reaction. Certainly, the individual's constitution must play some role in any reaction.

WATSON: The reason for a reaction depends on the vaccine. Extensive testing is done on vaccines these days. In the case of whole-cell DTP, the reaction is an immune response to the whole organism. In the case of APDT (which has specific proteins), it is a reaction to the pertussis toxoid. As new vaccines are produced by molecular biologic technology, there is less chance of reacting to the culture medium, which was the case in the old duck embryo rabies vaccines, for instance. Reactions to additives and preservatives depend on the individual and are extremely rare. As with anything we expose our bodies to, be it food, drugs, or vaccines, the individual's immune response is likely to be unique.

12. CAN PARENTS ANTICIPATE OR EVALUATE THEIR CHILD'S RISK OF REACTION TO VACCINE?

CASTRO: This is unfortunately (and sometimes tragically) hard to predict. Perfectly healthy children can and do suffer serious reactions to vaccination. To a certain extent, the health of the child can be used as a measure, i.e., a healthy child is more likely to cope better with immunizations than one who is unwell, especially one with a compromised immune system or a history of recurring, chronic complaints. A history of adverse vaccine reactions in either or both of the parents should be taken into account. Allergies, asthma, hay fever, or eczema in the personal or family history can be indications that a child is at a higher risk than those with good health.

MONTGOMERY: Other than avoiding vaccines that have components to which the child is allergic, I would have to say that it is difficult to predict the risks for the first vaccine in a series. If a child reacts to a dose of vaccine, he or she is likely to have a similar reaction to subsequent doses.

MOSKOWITZ: Yes, to some extent. A history of bad reactions in older siblings or from a previous dose is a definite warning. Many of Coulter and Fisher's (the authors of *DPT: A Shot in the Dark*) most gruesome cases of brain-injured infants had reacted badly to early DPT shots, but their pediatricians had ignored these warnings and insisted on continuing the series.

WATSON: Giving a full family history to the pediatrician is the best service a parent can do.

13. HOW CAN A PARENT TELL IF A CHILD HAS HAD A REACTION TO A VACCINE? WHAT SYMPTOMS SHOULD A PARENT LOOK FOR? OVER WHAT PERIOD OF TIME? WHAT CAN PARENTS DO IF THEY SUSPECT THAT THEIR CHILD HAS HAD A REACTION TO A VACCINE OR IS AT RISK FOR ONE?

CASTRO: If the child is different in any way (if any aspect of his or her behavior is altered) after a vaccine, then he or she has reacted to it and should be watched closely. Careful notes should be kept (including the date and time of the vaccine and all reactions) and medical professionals informed.

Local reactions at the site of the vaccination should be monitored but are rarely a cause for concern. These include inflammation (swelling and redness). Sometimes these form painful, hard lumps that can last for several weeks or even months. Parents should be on the lookout for the following general reactions: crying, in particular a high-pitched crying that might indicate brain damage; restlessness; unresponsiveness (in children who were formerly lively); excessive sleepiness; any alterations in sleep or appetite; or fever.

Long-term reactions are more difficult to evaluate. Parents will find it useful to take note of any increase in acute illnesses such as ear infections, sore throats, and coughs; developmental delay; skin rashes; and allergies or breathing difficulties.

Local reactions take place immediately and should be gone within a few days. General reactions usually occur immediately (within a week) and can last days, weeks, or may sometimes be permanent. Long-term, chronic reactions are more variable with regard to when they appear and can occur weeks or even months after vaccination.

Parents need to keep careful notes if they suspect a reaction so they can inform healthcare professionals. These notes may also be helpful in their future decisions about vaccination. If a child has reacted badly to a particular vaccine, the chances of a similar (or worse) reaction with subsequent vaccinations are high. Homeopathic treatment has proven effective in treating children suffering from a wide range of side effects (immediate and long-term) of vaccinations. Some parents who have chosen to vaccinate their children routinely take them for a constitutional remedy afterward to boost their immune system and minimize the risk of side effects. Vaccines should be delayed or not given if the child has one or more of the following: a fever; any acute infection (however mild), including colds, earache, and so forth; a chronic disease of any sort, i.e., if the immune system is weak; allergies; a history of convulsions; developmental delay.

MONTGOMERY: Generally, for live virus vaccines, the time period is similar to that for the natural infection, usually seven to 15 days for the common viruses (MMR, varicella). For polio, up to 30 hours is reportable for a person with a normal immune system. Cases of paralytic polio in immunocompromised people are reportable for up to six months after administration. For the inactivated viruses, any reactions are going to occur within the first few days and not after more than about a week.

If parents suspect their child has had a reaction to a vaccine, they should notify the healthcare provider who administered the vaccine. The provider may want to make changes in the schedule or, in the case of pertussis, eliminate the vaccine from the next dose. All significant adverse reactions should be reported by the provider to the Vaccine Adverse Event Reporting System. For milder reactions, such as fever and fussiness, it is prudent to give acetaminophen before vaccination.

MOSKOWITZ: Many of the commoner reactions are difficult to detect because they are simply aggravations of whatever tendencies were already there. In newborns and young infants, detecting them may be even more difficult because they represent their very first immunological experiences. Apart from the obvious immediate reactions, such as fever, local swelling, fussiness, and the like, many parents report that their kid has never been the same since a certain vaccine, or notice definite personality or behavior changes, developmental delays, or increases in common diseases (ear infections, asthma, and so forth).

14. WHAT LESSONS CAN WE LEARN FROM OTHER COUNTRIES REGARDING THE BENEFITS AND RISKS OF VACCINES?

GORDON: We can learn from England's experience with suspension of the pertussis vaccine. Either the number of pertussis cases actually went up, or doctors just decided to report a lot more whooping cough. Probably mostly the former and a little of the latter occurred.

MONTGOMERY: For one thing, pharmaceutical laws tend to be less restrictive in other countries, so most things are studied there earlier. For example, the acellular pertussis vaccine studies are coming out of Japan and Europe. This restrictiveness of our FDA has advantages and disadvantages; we can be pretty sure that things available here have been very well studied, but it also takes a lot longer for us to have access to them.

We can study the variations in disease occurrence by vaccination rate; some countries have nearly full vaccination, and many have higher vaccination rates than the US. In countries with low rates of vaccination, we are reminded of the often devastating effects of epidemics of vaccine-preventable diseases. Several outbreaks in other industrialized countries have occurred in recent years that give us information about the importance of high vaccination rates and also about the continued threat of some of these diseases.

Two deaths related to pertussis vaccine but not caused by it occurred in Japan in 1975, and the ministry of health suspended pertussis vaccination for two months. Many parents subsequently chose not to vaccinate against pertussis, and the vaccination rate dropped. From 1971 to 1974, there were less than 400 cases annually in Japan and only ten pertussis deaths in that period. From 1975 to 1979, there were 113 deaths; more than 13,000 cases were reported in 1979. In England, because of similar concerns about vaccine safety, the vaccination rate for pertussis dropped from about 75 percent to about 25 percent in the mid-1970s. From 1977 to 1979, a major pertussis epidemic occurred. Forty deaths from pertussis were reported, and increased death rates from "pneumonia" in the period probably represented undiagnosed pertussis deaths as well. Sweden stopped pertussis vaccination in 1979; it has had major outbreaks in 1982, 1983, and 1985.

Polio outbreaks occurred among groups who refused immunization on religious grounds in the Netherlands, Canada, and the US in 1978 and 1979 but did not spread beyond the unimmunized groups. On the other hand, an outbreak of polio in Finland in 1984 and 1985 led to nine cases of paralytic polio. Lab and sewage analysis led to the estimate of 100,000 people infected, despite high levels of IPV immunization in the community. The outbreak was controlled with a focused program of OPV immunization. The virus was determined to be a slightly different strain of wild poliovirus.

15. WHAT WOULD YOU ADVISE REGARDING TRAVEL AND VACCINES?

CASTRO: My advice is to have the minimum number of vaccines (as opposed to the maximum often recommended by travel agents, doctors, and airlines). Contact the embassy of the country concerned and ask about the legal requirements and the prevalence of current diseases. Make sure that the vaccination program is completed at least six weeks before departure. This will give the immune system a chance to recover before the stresses of traveling (especially if it is to a high-risk country). And if there are any adverse reactions, they can be dealt with at home rather than having the child fall sick while on vacation.

If two or more vaccinations are required, have them done one at a time, with a gap of two weeks between each shot. This enables the body to deal with the stress of vaccination more effectively. Certain areas are high risk with regard to epidemic diseases (South America, Asia, and certain parts of Africa), and some parents choose to avoid them. If your child is at risk from vaccines because of a previous history of adverse reactions or because of a compromised immune system, you might want to consider traveling to a low-risk country.

GORDON: Asia, Africa, some parts of the Caribbean, and other parts of the world have more disease and poorer health than we have in North America. Travel to India or Africa may put one at risk for polio, diphtheria, and other diseases we have little or no experience with in the US. Families who travel a lot should vaccinate against these and other illnesses. Most of the additional vaccines—cholera, yellow fever, and others—have side effects that make me want to consider them on a case-by-case basis only. The new vaccine for hepatitis A (transmitted by "food handlers") is worth at least a second thought. It may save more than a few vacations from ending with a bad illness.

WATSON: When traveling to areas where there are diseases rarely seen in the US—such as polio, measles, mumps, yellow fever, pertussis, diphtheria, and tetanus—it is essential to protect the child. Traveling unprotected to countries where these diseases are still common is like allowing a baby to play with a loaded gun. Would I suggest that parents reconsider vaccines or consider additional ones when traveling outside their home country? Absolutely.

MOSKOWITZ: Evaluate each vaccine individually according to the risk and efficacy of the vaccine and the prevalence and severity of the disease. Remember that selective use of a vaccine for short-term protection in a healthy child or adult is very different from bombarding a newborn infant with multiple vaccines purely as a matter of policy.

Thus, if I were contemplating a long period of residence in a country where yellow fever is rampant, I might well choose to be vaccinated. Cholera and typhoid vaccines, on the other hand, are much less effective, and good treatments are available for these diseases. Polio, diphtheria, and tetanus are still prevalent in many developing countries, and these vaccines might be worth considering for anybody living there for a long time, except perhaps nursing infants under two years of age.

16. CAN WE AFFORD FREEDOM OF CONSCIENCE REGARDING VACCINATIONS IN THE UNITED STATES? IN THE WORLD?

CASTRO: Can Americans afford *not* to have freedom of conscience with regard to vaccinations? It is the unalienable right of the

American individual, as I understand it, to stand up for what he or she believes is right and true. I have seen this in operation in many areas and walks of life in this country and admire it enormously.

Vaccinations have never been publicly debated in any country in the world. The vaccination program is, in effect, a mass medical intervention on the part of a medical establishment dedicated to eradicating epidemic diseases. The intention is good, but because the efficacy and safety of immunizations have been called into question, a public debate is necessary (with both sides presenting their cases) so that parents can make an informed choice. Parents have a right to make an educated decision, to resist mass medication if they so choose—for themselves and/or their children. It has been hard to evaluate the risks because parents are coerced into immunizing their children without adequate information.

GORDON: Not vaccinating your children may be regarded as a selfish act. An intelligently considered selfish act—but selfish nonetheless. On the other hand, if we're not going to be selfish about our children, when will we ever be selfish? No, we probably cannot afford "freedom of conscience" when we promote vaccinations in underdeveloped countries: If we stop vaccinating, the rate of infectious diseases could increase precipitously, leading to millions of preventable deaths in children and adults.

MONTGOMERY: This is a very difficult question for me to answer. I would hate to think that we could not afford freedom of conscience on any question. The answer depends on what risks we wish to take as individuals and as a society. Is it worth the slight increase in risk of outbreaks if a small percentage of the population remains unvaccinated in a country where disease is uncommon? Probably, since freedom is such a closely held value here. Is it worth risking the deaths of thousands of children if entire countries or regions fail to implement vaccine programs? I don't think so. I feel it is important for us to have vaccine policy throughout the world so that the majority of people are vaccinated and the diseases can be controlled or eliminated, but that individual parents can and should make informed decisions about how they will apply that policy to their own children.

Another factor in this equation is the growing number of diseases for which we have no cure. Viruses such as herpes and HIV can be treated but not cured with antiviral drugs. Many bacteria are developing resistance to some or all antibiotics. After a half-century of believing that we could develop drugs to cure all infectious diseases, we are moving into the "post-antibiotic era." I believe that vaccines will be an even more essential part of a strategy to control infectious diseases in the future, as one component of the effort to prevent disease rather than try to treat it once it's there. People will still have to make thoughtful choices, but the stakes will be getting higher.

WATSON: No. Any unimmunized individual is at risk. Additionally, unimmunized individuals serve as reservoirs for disease, which can then be spread to infants too young to be immunized and to people with compromised immune systems. The US is not an island, with more than a million visitors from Asia and Africa each year. We should have JFK's vision that ridding the world of disease is as important as ridding the world of wars. When you make a decision not to immunize your child, you are possibly affecting the fate of others, as well.

MOSKOWITZ: Lacking adequate studies of their long-term health risks, we are reckless indeed to require universal vaccination of all children against the wishes of their parents and in the absence of a genuine public-health emergency. At present, almost half the states allow parents to waive the vaccination requirement on the basis of their personal conviction, i.e., if they are prepared to withstand the social opprobrium of being seen as a kook. No state yet authorizes parents to make an intelligent medical decision for their kids by accepting some vaccines but not others, as is already common practice in Europe and elsewhere. Can we afford not to give our citizens the same freedom of conscience enjoyed by most of the civilized world? I don't think so.

17. HOW DO YOU HELP THE PARENTS WITH WHOM YOU WORK SORT OUT THE CONFLICTING INFORMATION REGARDING VACCINATIONS? WHAT ADVICE CAN YOU GIVE TO PARENTS REGARDING THE VACCINATION DECISION?

CASTRO: The responsibility of parents confronted with an issue that affects their child's well-being is the same as with any other intervention (medical or otherwise): to protect their child from harm, to make an informed and educated decision. This decision-making process may be challenging and even troubling for doctors and parents, but it needs addressing so that parents can be active participants in decisions that affect their children's welfare. Parents have to somehow evaluate whether vaccination represents a significant threat to their child's health, in which case they may decide not to have their child vaccinated. Or they may decide that vaccinations will help their children to ward off epidemic diseases and choose to have all the vaccinations that are available. Or they may fall somewhere in between, seeing the benefits of certain vaccines but being concerned about the risks with others, especially those in which the risks from the disease are minimal. These parents may decide that some immunizations are unnecessary or risky, while others are valuable enough to choose them for their children.

GORDON: Parents must arm themselves with as much information as possible, with the knowledge that this is a polarized issue with virtually nobody telling the whole truth. What it boils down to is the fact that there are some risks involved in getting vaccines and some risks in not being vaccinated. The risks on both sides of the coin are probably very small, and it is up to each individual family to take a responsible, intelligent look at the issue.

MONTGOMERY: I consider myself generally provaccination but respectful of parental choice. I believe parents must look at their children's health from an overall perspective and try to enhance their disease-fighting ability in each area. They also need to make choices that fit their family's values and needs.

Clearly, healthy kids have a much better chance of avoiding disease and/or having milder disease. Growing healthy kids involves good nutrition, starting with breastfeeding and continuing with it for a long time. It also involves hygiene. Psychological well-being is probably more essential to a healthy immune system than traditional medicine has recognized in the past, although we are catching on. People are pretty much designed to be exposed to smaller family or clan groups, so limiting exposure to large numbers of children from different families will decrease the risk of exposure to diseases. (It is true, however, that kids who are in daycare and get sick a lot when they are younger tend to get sick less often by the time they get to kindergarten.) Parents who are home with their children and/or who homeschool may have different concerns about kids having a long illness, such as pertussis or chickenpox, than those who would need to miss work to care for their children or whose children would miss long stretches of school.

When I counsel parents about vaccines, I generally recommend that they follow the immunizations schedule unless they have specific concerns or objections. I give all parents as much information as I can about the diseases and the vaccines so they can make an informed choice. For those who are determined not to vaccinate at all, I try to be sure they are fully informed of the risks of the diseases and explore with them their reasons for not vaccinating. If I am comfortable that they are making an informed choice not to vaccinate, I do not push them to do otherwise. If parents are concerned about the number of vaccines given all at once, I work with them to develop a vaccine schedule that fits their family. (In my own case, I felt that hepatitis B was not an immediate risk for my son, so I delayed that vaccination while giving him the others on schedule.) If parents are concerned primarily about side effects, I encourage them to give the safer vaccines for disease that occur in infancy, such as Hib, on schedule and delay some of the others until they are comfortable. In the case of pertussis, the acellular vaccine can be given after age 18 months; some parents may wish to delay DTP until then.

As with any choices they make for their children, parents should try to get all the information they can about vaccines and evaluate it as objectively as possible. I have little patience for dogmatic approaches either for or against vaccinations. As I have tried to indicate, each disease for which we have a vaccine is unique, and each vaccine has unique properties. I don't find it very useful to lump them and say "all vaccines are wonderful" or "all vaccines are terrible." Vaccines have done a great deal of good in preventing illness and death, but they are not perfect. Some are clearly better than others. Vaccine science has come a long way but still has further to go. Many improvements are coming along in vaccines. Parents who have chosen not to vaccinate or to delay vaccination should stay informed about new developments and reevaluate their choices on an ongoing basis.

WATSON: I present scientific data and educate parents about the disease process and the immune response. As someone who has been a general pediatrician and family physician for 20 years, an infectious disease specialist for 14 years in three countries (including an African one), and has been involved in vaccine research for eight years, I have seen many children suffer and die from the ravages of vaccine-preventable diseases. I have not yet seen a child suffer permanent injury or death as a result of immunizations. My message to parents is as follows: The diseases are real, they are dangerous, and they are a threat to our children. Do not rely on those around you to protect your child from disease by immunizing their children. Parents need to be fully informed about the relative benefits and risks of any treatment or preventative measure so that they can make the best decision on behalf of their child.

DISEASE RISKS

RUBELLA

GREATEST # CASES	SYMPTOMS	
57,686 20,000 Congenital Rubella Syndrome (1964–1965)	Very mild, slight fever; faint pink rash; swelling of neck, underarm, and groin glands	
	LENGTH OF DISEASE: 3 days	INCUBATION PERIOD: 14–21 days
	INFECTIOUS PERIOD: 5 days before and 7 days after rash appears; stay away from pregnant women	

1992 CASES	COMPLICATIONS	DEATH RATE
148 Rubella 9 Congenital Rubella Syndrome	Joint swelling in adult women 1:3 (onset 1–2 weeks) Purpura (temporary bleeding disorder) 1:6,000 Encephalitis 1:6,000 Miscarriage or birth defects in pregnant women 1.7:100,000 (60 infants per year)	1:5,000

DIPHTHERIA

GREATEST # CASES	SYMPTOMS	
206,939 (1921)	Infection characterized by the formation of a fake membrane on any mucous surface and occasionally on the skin	

1992 CASES	COMPLICATIONS	DEATH RATE
4	Infection can interfere with breathing Heart failure Paralysis	1:10

TETANUS

GREATEST # CASES	SYMPTOMS	
1,560 (1923)	Serious painful spasms of all muscles caused by poison of tetanus bacteria in infected wound	

1992 CASES	COMPLICATIONS	DEATH RATE
42	Lockjaw Death	4:10

VACCINATION RISKS AND BENEFITS

MMR

PERCENT EFFECTIVE 90% if not vaccinated before 15 months

SIDE EFFECTS OF VACCINE; ONSET OF SIDE EFFECTS

Mild swelling of neck glands and rash (probably of rubella component) 1:7 (onset: 1–2 weeks)

Few days of joint aching or swelling 1:100 (onset: 1–3 weeks)

Adult temporary joint swelling 1:40

Arthritis 1:50

Rash, slight fever 1:6.5–1:20 (onset: 48 hours–2 weeks)

Anaphylaxis or anaphylactic shock; extremely rare (onset: 24 hours)

Encephalitis 1:2,500,000 (onset: 15 days)

POSSIBLE CONTRAINDICATIONS TO VACCINE

Moderate or severe illness	Medication that reduces resistance to infection
Previous severe reaction to MMR vaccine	Pregnancy (rubella)
Severe allergic reaction to egg protein	Seizure (mumps)
Cancer	Sibling or parent who has had a seizure (mumps)
Leukemia (rubella)	Immune globulin or transfusion in last few months (rubella)
Lymphoma (rubella)	

DT DPT(DTP) TD DTAP

PERCENT EFFECTIVE 95% DT only

SIDE EFFECTS OF VACCINE; ONSET OF SIDE EFFECTS

Soreness

Slight fever (onset: 24 hours)

POSSIBLE CONTRAINDICATIONS TO VACCINE

Moderate or severe illness

Previous severe reaction to vaccine

DT DPT DTP DTAP TD

PERCENT EFFECTIVE T: 95%

SIDE EFFECTS OF VACCINE; ONSET OF SIDE EFFECTS

Soreness

Slight fever (onset: 24 hours)

POSSIBLE CONTRAINDICATIONS TO VACCINE

Moderate or severe illness

Previous severe reaction to vaccine

Disease Risks

MUMPS		
GREATEST # CASES	SYMPTOMS	
152,209 (1968)	Fever, headache, inflammation of salivary glands and possibly glands under tongue and jaw, causing cheeks to swell LENGTH OF DISEASE: 1–2 weeks INCUBATION PERIOD: 12–28 days INFECTIOUS PERIOD: 2 days before swelling appears until swelling subsides	
1992 CASES	COMPLICATIONS	DEATH RATE
2,460	Mild meningitis 1:10 Deafness 6:100 Encephalitis 4:100 (onset: 15 days) Painful testicle inflammation in adolescent or adult males 1:4 Sterility in adolescent or adult males—rare	1–3:10,000

MEASLES		
GREATEST # CASES	SYMPTOMS	
894,134 (1941)	Small spots like grains of sand in mouth and inside cheeks (Koplick's spots); rash—blotchy, itchy, with raised spots; high fever; runny nose; red, watery eyes sensitive to light LENGTH OF DISEASE: 1–2 weeks INCUBATION PERIOD: 18–21 days INFECTIOUS PERIOD: 4 days before and 5–10 days after rash appears	
1992 CASES	COMPLICATIONS	DEATH RATE
2,200	Ear infection 1:10 Pneumonia 1:10 Encephalitis (can lead to convulsions, deafness, and mental retardation) 1:1,000	1:5,000

Vaccination Risks and Benefits

MMR

Percent Effective 90% if not vaccinated before 15 months

Side Effects of Vaccine; Onset of Side Effects

Occasional mild swelling of salivary glands (probably of mumps component), rash, slight fever 1:6.5–1:20 (onset: 48 hours–2 weeks)

Anaphylaxis or anaphylactic shock; extremely rare (onset: 24 hours)

Encephalitis 1:2,500,000 (onset: 15 days)

Possible Contraindications to Vaccine

Moderate or severe illness	Medication that reduces resistance to infection
Previous reaction to MMR vaccine	
Severe allergic reaction to egg protein	Pregnancy (rubella)
	Seizure (mumps)
Cancer	Sibling or parent who has had a seizure (mumps)
Leukemia (rubella)	
Lymphoma (rubella)	Immune globulin or transfusion in last few months (rubella)

MMR

Percent Effective 90% if not vaccinated before 15 months

Side Effects of Vaccine; Onset of Side Effects

Rash, slight fever 1:6.5–1:20 (onset: 48 hours–2 weeks)

Anaphylaxis or anaphylactic shock; extremely rare (onset: 24 hours)

Encephalitis 1:2,500,000 (onset: 15 days)

Possible Contraindications to Vaccine

Moderate or severe illness	Medication that reduces resistance to infection
Previous reaction to MMR vaccine	
Severe allergic reaction to egg protein	Pregnancy (rubella)
	Seizure (mumps)
Cancer	Sibling or parent who has had a seizure (mumps)
Leukemia (rubella)	
Lymphoma (rubella)	Immune globulin or transfusion in last few months (rubella)

Disease Risks

Hemophilus Influenzae Type b Meningitis

Greatest # Cases	Symptoms	
12,000 (1987) (50% 1 year or under)	Cold, ear infection, lethargy, bulging fontanel, neck stiffness, eating difficulty, infection of the covering of the brain	

1993 Cases	Complications	Death Rate
17	Moderate to severe cases under 5 years old (serious in those under 1 year old) 1:200 Pneumonia Infections of blood, joints, bone, soft tissue, under skin, throat, and covering of the heart Permanent brain damage 1:4 Deafness 1:4	1:20

Sources for Risks/Benefits Charts

Castro, Miranda. "Childhood Diseases at a Glance." *Mothering* 77 (Winter 1995): 37.

"Comparison of Incidence of Risks and Complications between the Disease of Pertussis Versus the DPT Vaccine," *Advances in Pediatric Diseases* 6 (1991): 1–55.

Giles, Vicki. "Vaccination and Individual Freedom." In *Vaccinations: The Rest of the Story*, edited by Peggy O'Mara. Santa Fe, NM: *Mothering Magazine*, 1992.

Lederle Biological Trial Data. Use of APDT in Infants. Publication pending.

Mortimer, Edward, and Stanley Plotkin, eds. "Vaccines and Toxoids, Adverse Events, and Intervals from Vaccinations to Onset of Adverse Event Required for Reporting or Compensation, United States" and "Comparison of Maximum and Current Morbidity and Vaccine-Peventable Diseases." In *Vaccines*, 2nd ed. Philadelphia: W. B. Saunders, 1994.

US Department of Health and Human Services. Centers for Disease Control and Prevention, *Hemophilus b Conjugate Vaccine, DTP, MMR, and Polio* (10 July 1995).

Vaccination Risks and Benefits

Hemophilus b Conjugate (not necessary for children over 5 or adults)

Percent Effective 90%

Side Effects of Vaccine; Onset of Side Effects

Fever above 101° 1:50 (onset: 24–48 hours)

Redness and swelling at site of injection 1:100 (onset: 24–48 hours)

Possible Contraindications to Vaccine

Moderate or severe illness

Serious reaction to thimersal, a mercurial antiseptic included in one vaccine

Serious allergic reaction to vaccine containing diphtheria toxoid

UNDERSTANDING THE POLIO VACCINE
BY ANNE MONTGOMERY

Poliomyelitis virus causes a range of symptoms, from a relatively mild disease to full-blown paralytic polio. Epidemics of polio continued until the mid-1950s in the US. The first polio vaccine, an inactivated vaccine, was introduced in 1955. This caused a significant decrease in the incidence of polio but did not eliminate it. There are three serotypes ("strains") of wild polio-virus; the body's first line of defense is in the gut. The oral polio vaccine (OPV), introduced in 1963, had the significant advantage of providing immunity to all three serotypes, and of providing gastrointestinal as well as serologic immunity to polio. Since it is oral rather than injectable, adminstration and mass immunization are much easier. The incidence of polio dropped even more dramatically after introduction of the oral polio vaccine, and wild-virus polio has been eliminated from the Western Hemisphere, with global elimination a possibility in the not too distant future. A newer, more effective inactivated polio vaccine (IPV) was introduced in 1987, but it still does not provide gastrointestinal immunity and is an injection; however, it is safer than the oral vaccine because it cannot cause vaccine-related disease.

Unlike other live virus vaccines, oral polio vaccine is given in several doses beginning in early infancy. Maternal serologic antibody to polio does not interfere with immunization (as it can with measles) and also provides less protection from polio than from other diseases. Several doses are required because the three serotypes can interfere with each other. By giving three doses plus a booster, we can obtain immunity to all three serotypes nearly 100 percent of the time. Theoretically, there should be polio IgA in breastmilk. Of course the introduction of the oral polio vaccine corresponded to the nadir of breastfeeding in this country, and now with no wild virus around, it is impossible to study the effect of breastfeeding as protection from polio in infancy in the US.

The major concern now with the polio vaccine is the risk of vaccine-associated paralytic polio. IPV should be given to all immunocompromised children and to all children who have an immunocompromised household contact. Any adult who has not had a polio vaccine should receive a dose of IPV before receiving OPV. Adults should be immunized before traveling to endemic areas and should

DISEASE RISKS

PARALYTIC POLIOMYELITIS

GREATEST # CASES	SYMPTOMS	
21,269 (1952)	Viral disease with flulike symptoms	

1992 CASES	COMPLICATIONS	DEATH RATE
0 Last natural polio in US in 1979 Last case in Americas in Peru in 1991 5–10 vaccine related cases	Permanent crippling Occasional death	76% (in children under 2) 7% (in those over 2)

VACCINATION RISKS AND BENEFITS

ORAL POLIO VACCINE
OPV
IPV
eIPV SALK INACTIVATED WITH FORMALIN

PERCENT EFFECTIVE OPV: 90% • IPV Salk: 80% (4–5 doses) • eIPV: 95% (3 doses)

SIDE EFFECTS OF VACCINE; ONSET OF SIDE EFFECTS

Vaccine-associated paralysis 1:520,000; first dose

1:12,300,000–1:18,000,000 subsequent doses

10% of all vaccine-associated paralysis in immunodeficient recipients

(onset for three effects listed above: 30 hours in nonimmunodeficient recipient; 6 months in immunodeficient recipient)

Anaphylaxis or anaphylactic shock is a rare reaction to any vaccine

POSSIBLE CONTRAINDICATIONS TO VACCINE

Moderate to severe illness
Previous serious reaction to OPV or IPV vaccine
Immunosuppressed or living with someone who is
Pregnant
Allergy to neomycin or streptomycin
(OPV only)
On long-term steroids
Cancer
Radiation therapy
AIDS or HIV

be immunized before their children start receiving OPV. If another person in the family/household has not been previously vaccinated, she or he should receive IPV vaccine before the infant begins the OPV series. Ideally, he or she should receive one dose when the baby is born and a second one month later, with the child beginning the OPV series at two months of age.

With the newer, more effective IPV available, there is a growing push for a change in polio vaccination policy, which I think we will see very soon. The next step will be to start giving IPV as the first polio immunization to reduce the risk of later vaccine-associated polio, followed by OPV to complete the series because of its greater immunogenicity and ease of administration. Once wild-virus polio is eradicated from the world, or nearly eradicated so that travel-related spread is unlikely, IPV will probably replace OPV for a time. Once all vaccine-related polio is eliminated, we will be able to stop vaccinating against polio (as we have done with smallpox).

The Advisory Committee on Immunization Practices (ACIP) recently voted to recommend that polio vaccination series consist of two doses of eIPV followed by two doses of OPV (in place of the current four-dose OPV series at two, four, six months, and preschool). CDC approval is likely but still pending.

WEIGHING THE FACTS ABOUT PERTUSSIS
BY JAY GORDON

Whooping cough (pertussis) is a serious disease that can be fatal in very young children. Pertussis may last six to ten weeks and is particularly dangerous in the first year of life. Of the children under one year of age who contract whooping cough—approximately half of all reported cases—about 20 percent get pneumonia, and 1 to 3 percent of all cases are complicated by seizures or other neurological involvement. Under six months of age, the mortality rate is quoted at .05 to 1 percent. The occurrence rate in Los Angeles County is reported to be between 300 and 500 cases per year.

The disease is usually caught from older siblings or adults. You can carry whooping cough asymptomatically, but this is not common. Pertussis is probably most contagious during pre-coughing days but may last as long as three weeks; erythromycin shortens the contagious period to less than a week. Laboratory tests for pertussis are not always reliable and usually are falsely negative by the time the cough is truly noticed as "pertussoid" in nature—that is, paroxysmal, staccato, sometimes followed by a "whoop." Not all "whooping" coughs are pertussis, however, and many children with pertussis do not whoop.

Treatment consists of erythromycin for two weeks, isolation for five days with antibiotics, or three weeks without antibiotics. After five days on erythromycin, a child may return to school, daycare, or play groups.

You now know much more about pertussis than you ever may have desired, but the decision about whether or not to give the vaccine to your child still may not be clear because you know that the other side of the issue is supported by strong, published medical facts. According to the "Report of the Committee on Infectious Diseases of the American Academy of Pediatrics" (1991), half of the children receiving this vaccine are reported to be "fretful," and/or have fevers. Severe neurological problems (brain damage or death) are reported in one in 140,000 to one in 310,000 children. Seizures are reported in one in 1,750 vaccine recipients. Persistent screaming for three or more hours is noted in one in 100 shots, and an unusual, high-pitched cry is a one in 1,000 complication.

The disease is bad, and the vaccine is far from perfect. In coun-

DISEASE RISKS

PERTUSSIS

GREATEST # CASES	SYMPTOMS	
265,269 (1934)	Begins with slight fever, runny nose, and loose cough. Can develop severe coughing spells that interfere with eating, drinking, and breathing. **LENGTH OF DISEASE:** 3–12 weeks **INCUBATION PERIOD:** 7–21 days **INFECTIOUS PERIOD:** 3–4 weeks following appearance of illness	
1992 CASES	**COMPLICATIONS**	**DEATH RATE**
3,359 (70% in children under 5)	*(In infants under 6 months)* Hospitalized 3:4 Intensive Care 1:20 Pneumonia 1:5 Scleral hemorrhage and epistaxis 1:5 Convulsions 1:40 Encephalopathy 1:240	1:100

VACCINATION RISKS AND BENEFITS

DPT DTP DTaP

PERCENT EFFECTIVE P: 36–83% (depending on manufacturer and country studied)   aP: 84–95% (depending on manufacturer)

SIDE EFFECTS OF VACCINE; ONSET OF SIDE EFFECTS

Soreness and swelling at site of injection. Slight fever and irritability—1:2 (onset: 24–48 hours)

Temperature above 102°—DTP 1:25; DTaP 1:50 (onset: 24–48 hours)

Temperature above 105°—DTP 1:333; DTaP 1:500 (onset: 24–48 hours)

Persistent cry—DTP 1:100; DTaP 1:100

Unusual high-pitched cry—DTP 1:100; DTaP 1:100–1:250

Limpness and pallor—DTP 1:1,667; DTaP 0

Convulsions—DTP 1:1,667; DTaP 0

Severe brain problem 1:10,000

Encephalopathy 1:100,000 (onset: 3–7 days)

Permanent brain damage 1:310,000

Anaphylaxis or anaphylactic shock (onset: 24 hours); rare

Shock-collapse or hyporesponse or hypotonic response (onset: 3–7 days); rare

Residual seizure disorder (onset: 3 days); rare

POSSIBLE CONTRAINDICATIONS TO VACCINE

Moderate to severe illness

Previous serious reaction to DTP, DPT, or DTaP shot

Undiagnosed seizures

Sibling or parent who has had a seizure or has had a serious reaction to DTP, DPT, or DTaP shot

Brain problem or central nervous system problem

tries where the vaccination rate for pertussis was greatly decreased, the disease and its complications increased dramatically. The vaccine does not always confer complete immunity; in some studies a significant percentage of the children with pertussis had been completely vaccinated. Partial vaccination does seem to lessen the severity of the disease. Still, "half-dose" vaccines seem to have the risk of a full dose without giving the benefits.

There are official reasons not to give a child this vaccine: a severe reaction to a prior vaccine, which may include a convulsion, the screaming syndrome, a temperature of 105° or higher, or an immediate, severe allergic reaction to a prior vaccine. A history of prior neurological disorders of a stable or unstable nature or a personal history of seizures requires a very careful balancing of risks and rewards in each individual child.

I do not feel that you are taking a large risk by giving your child the complete DPT (diphtheria-pertussis-tetanus) vaccine. I also do not feel that you are taking a large risk by omitting the "P" and just giving the diphtheria-tetanus alternative. Conversely, I think that either choice carries a small statistical risk.

The above opinions make it obvious that a decision is very difficult, but virtually all experts and other pediatricians recommend in favor of vaccinating all children who do not fall into the categories mentioned above. My opposition to unbridled enthusiasm for this vaccine is tempered by the knowledge that a change in national vaccination policy would be dangerous, and we may be forced to accept a small number of children having severe complications in the best interests of the pediatric population as a whole.

The New DTP: DTaP
By Anne Montgomery

One of the most interesting developments in vaccine policy will be the shift from the standard DPT with the whole-cell pertussis vaccine to the DTaP with the acellular pertussis vaccine for the primary series in infants. This vaccine is currently licensed for use for the 18-month and pre-kindergarten booster but has not yet been used in the US because of concerns about its efficacy in younger children. Recent studies in Sweden and Italy have shown the acellular vaccine to be as effective, if not more effective, than the whole-cell vaccine. Studies are still ongoing to determine the appropriate number of doses and whether combination vaccines, including DTaP with Hib and other vaccines, will also be effective. A license application was submitted in July 1995, and the acellular vaccine is approved for infants now. This vaccine does not completely eliminate the problems with the pertussis vaccine but should decrease the side effects fairly significantly. DTaP should not be given to children who have had a serious reaction to DTP.

Vaccines are being studied for herpes, HIV, and several other diseases. The pneumococcal vaccine may prove useful in children, particularly if a protein conjugate vaccine such as Hib can be developed, as it could prevent many case of otitis media as well as pneumonia. As we move into the postantibiotic era, more and more vaccines will be developed. With improved technology and improved understanding of the immune system, the newer vaccines are likely to be more effective and safer than the older vaccines. Parents will need to evaluate each one as it comes along in order to make appropriate choices for their children.

TO VACCINATE OR NOT? A GUIDE FOR MAKING A CHOICE
BY MIRANDA CASTRO

Weigh the pros and cons of each vaccination, gathering information from both sides. It is sensible to do this when pregnant rather than wait until after the baby is born. (Parents are more vulnerable then and may find it hard to resist persuasion, however friendly.) Ideally, partners need to be involved in this decision-making process, too.

Parents should take their own beliefs and feelings into account when weighing the risk of contracting each disease versus the efficacy of each vaccination.

Seek out medical providers who are sympathetic to your needs and wishes. Parents deserve doctors sympathetic to their needs, especially their wish to make informed choices about every aspect of their child's health care, including vaccination.

Bear in mind that, as with any decision, you will have to live with the consequences. If you decide not to vaccinate, you will have to ask yourself whether you are prepared to nurse your child through a childhood illness such as measles or whooping cough or a more serious disease such as polio.

Likewise, you will also need to ask yourself how you might feel if your child contracted a particular disease from the vaccine or became chronically ill as a result of a vaccine program.

Wait as long as possible before you start your child's vaccination program.

Ask your doctor to administer one at a time; since we do not contract more than one disease at a time, it makes sense to have only one vaccine at a time. This way, if there is an adverse reaction, you and your doctor will know which one is the culprit.

Make your peace with the fact that this is a difficult decision and there are risks attached to any decision (whether you decide to vaccinate your child or not). Your goal is to make sure the risks are minimized.

THE VACCINATIONS

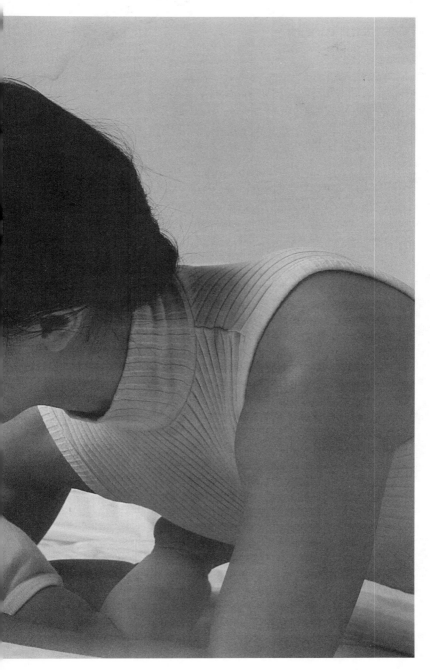

The MMR Vaccine
By Lynne McTaggart

Lynne McTaggart is an award-winning investigative journalist, author of several books, and editor of the newsletter What Doctors Don't Tell You. *She lives in London, England, with her husband, Bryan, and their daughter, Caitlin. "The MMR Vaccine" first appeared in* Mothering, *no. 63 (Spring 1992).*

My two-year-old daughter, Caitlin, and I are the targets of a £1.5 million ($2.7 million) advertising campaign. The British government and even my local health clinic are attempting to convince me to have her vaccinated against measles, mumps, and rubella (German measles).

Traditionally, the MMR campaign was restricted to physician handouts—brochures stating that the vaccine has for many years been used safely in other countries, particularly the US, and that it provides "lifelong protection against all three infections with a single jab." Now, emotive messages of all sorts are appearing in television ads depicting angelic, sleeping children.

Parents in the US are under similar pressure to give their children the live triple vaccine. The US government has suggested withholding welfare payments from any mother refusing to vaccinate her child. And Chicago health authorities have begun using loudspeaker sales pitches mixed with salsa music to encourage Hispanic mothers to take their children to neighborhood health clinics for shots.

A Spotty Take-Up Record

The recent fuss has come precisely because the vaccine appears not to be working. The US is witnessing a steadily increasing epidemic of measles—the worst in decades—even though the combined shot has been available since 1975 and the measles vaccine itself has been in effect since 1957. While the government-targeted date for elimination of the disease was set at 1982, the Centers for Disease Control (CDC) in Atlanta reported a provisional total of 27,672 cases of measles in 1990. This figure represents twice the amount reported in 1989, which was twice that reported in 1988.[1]

At first, the measles vaccine looked promising. The number of measles cases fell by 25 percent to 63,000 the year it was introduced.

After bottoming out at 1,500 in 1983, though, the number of cases swelled 423 percent by 1989 and is now sharply rising, especially in Houston, Texas, and Los Angeles County.[2]

The medical establishment blames the recent epidemic on clusters of unvaccinated children, especially those in poor, nonwhite neighborhoods. Statistics, however, prove otherwise. CDC data from 1989 shows that half of all college-age victims had been vaccinated. Moreover, between 1985 and 1986, two-thirds of all measles cases occurred in school-age children, the majority of whom had been vaccinated.[3]

"The appearance of measles is a sensitive indicator of the inadequacies of our vaccination system," announced Donald A. Henderson, chair of the National Vaccine Advisory Committee of the US Department of Health and Human Services, in tacit admission of the vaccine's failure. "It raises the specter of whether we might expect further down the line outbreaks of polio (should it be imported), pertussis and diphtheria."[4]

The epidemics occurring among college-age students are primarily affecting those born between 1957 and 1967, when the measles vaccine was introduced. The CDC currently estimates that between 5 and 15 percent of college students are susceptible.[5] As a result, students at many universities must provide proof of recent vaccination before registering for classes.

The problem, say CDC and other medical experts, is that the vaccine wears off in time, as does an individual's immunity. Others believe that those vaccinated between 1957 and 1980 received a less stable version of the vaccine than those who were vaccinated more recently. Consequently, experts in the US and elsewhere are recommending a variety of approaches: lowering the age of vaccination from 15 months to one year, or providing a measles booster shot at school age or later (around age 11) if the earlier booster has not been given, or administering the single measles shot at nine months and the combined shot at 15 months, or introducing the MMR at one year of age.

The American Academy of Pediatrics now recommends giving a second dose of MMR at age two. Still, some medics believe that not even two doses will be enough to deal with the "wild" strains of measles that have been appearing. Underlying all these "solutions" is the disquieting question: *Does it make sense to offer booster shots of any sort if a single shot of the vaccine has not been shown to do the job?*

Theories on vaccine ineffectiveness abound. According to some, shots are given too early, and their effectiveness is canceled out by maternal antibodies acquired in the womb. Others imply that the vaccine loses its potency if given when children have respiratory infections, or if the serum is improperly stored or handled.

The CDC estimates that up to 10 percent of all vaccinations do not take.[6] And indeed, study after study points unerringly to clusters of vaccinated children who have contracted measles. Here are just a few examples:

In a 1986 outbreak of measles in Corpus Christi, Texas, 99 percent of the children had been vaccinated and more than 95 percent were purportedly immune.[7]

In 1987, the CDC reported 2,440 cases of measles among vaccinated children. Forty-one percent of them had received the MMR vaccine between 12 and 14 months of age, and the remaining 59 percent had been vaccinated at 15 months or older.[8]

In 1985, 80 percent of all cases of measles in the US occurred in children who had been properly vaccinated at the appropriate age.[9]

Between 1985 and 1986, reports of measles outbreaks among school-age children revealed that 60 percent of them had been vaccinated.[10]

The rubella component of the vaccine has not fared well either. In the 1970s, Stanley Plotkin, MD, a professor of pediatrics at the University of Pennsylvania, evaluated adolescent girls who had received the vaccine during childhood. He found that more than one-third of them lacked any evidence of immunity against rubella.[11] More recently, an Italian study of 600 vaccinated girls showed that 10 percent of them had been infected by a wild strain of the virus—some within a few years of inoculation.[12]

DISEASE-RELATED COMPLICATIONS

The medical justification for the shots is that measles is a dangerous disease. Official statistics suggest that between one in 1,000 and one in 5,000 children who contract measles naturally—that is, not in response to the vaccine—will develop acute encephalitis (inflammation of the brain). Several years later, one in 5,000 of these youngsters will develop subacute sclerosing panencephalitis (SSPE), an often fatal progressive disease that causes hardening of the brain.[13]

The SSPE Registry report on the incidence of SSPE between 1960 and 1970, however, states that the measles-induced form of this disease is "very rare," occurring in one per million cases.[14] Furthermore, a study of 52 people with SSPE concludes that environmental factors other than measles, such as serious head injuries or close exposure to certain animals, contributed to the onset of disease. Researchers found "no differences with regard to the average age at vaccination, having received more than one measles vaccination, or having received measles vaccine after natural measles."[15]

Of the 89 suspected measles-associated deaths in the US in 1990, most occurred in low-income populations. Inadequate nutrition and poor living conditions played a part in the outcome, as did failure to treat complications.[16]

Childhood mumps and rubella, on the other hand, are ordinarily very mild illnesses, says Norman Begg, MD, consultant epidemiologist with the Public Health Laboratory Service, which recommended the triple vaccine in Britain. Mumps "very rarely" leads to long-term permanent complications, he notes. "On its own, mumps isn't a particularly cost-effective vaccine. But it provides extra benefit for the combined MMR vaccine."[17]

VACCINE-RELATED COMPLICATIONS

Risks are inherent in the vaccines themselves, and these appear far greater than the medical establishment claims. Moreover, complications are multiplied by a triple jab whose separate components carry individual risks.

According to the prevailing medical view, measles-vaccine-induced encephalitis is rare, occurring in one out of 200,000 children. Symptoms include fever, headache, possible convulsions, and behavioral changes. "Most symptoms are mild," Begg says, "and the children will recover."[18] The reported incidence of mumps-vaccine-induced meningitis is between one per 50,000 and one per million doses.[19]

Some studies using the same vaccine strains reveal significantly larger risks. A West German study places the incidence of reactions to the measles portion of the shot at one neurologic complication per 2,500 vaccinees and one case of temporary encephalitis per 17,650 vaccinees.[20] In several more recent studies, the measles vaccine strain recovered from victims' spines shows conclusively that the vaccine caused the encephalitis, says Dr. J. Anthony Morris, an immunization specialist formerly with the National Institutes of Health and the Food and Drug Administration.[21]

Of the first 10,000 British children given the measles vaccine, 2.5 per 1,000 suffered convulsions.[22] Wellcome, until recently one of three manufacturers of the MMR vaccine in Britain, reports that the measles portion of the vaccine may cause fever and rash, orchitis (inflammation of the testicle), nerve deafness, febrile convulsions, encephalitis, Guillain-Barré syndrome (a form of paralysis), SSPE, and atypical measles (marked by unusual symptoms).[23] In fact, the SSPE study cited above indicates that nearly one-third of all victims had received a measles vaccine prior to the onset of illness. "This study cannot confirm or rule out the possibility that the measles vaccine may lead to SSPE on rare occasions," the authors conclude.[24]

The mumps vaccine, too, is associated with complications. It is known to cause encephalitis, meningitis, seizures, unilateral nerve deafness, and other serious conditions. Researchers investigating all cases of mumps encephalitis over the previous 15 years concluded that one-sixth of them were due to the vaccine. "A recent increase appeared to be related to the introduction of a new mumps vaccine," they noted.[25] A Canadian study set the risk of mumps-vaccine-induced encephalitis at one per 100,000 recipients;[26] a Yugoslavian study at one per 1,000 recipients.[27]

Several physicians have written letters to *The Lancet* describing reactions to the mumps portion of the MMR vaccine. An Edinburgh doctor reported that a girl who had developed meningitis 21 days after the shot had the mumps virus strain isolated from her spinal fluid, and it matched the strain used in the vaccine.[28] A West German doctor wrote in to say that health authorities in his country had come up with 27 neurological reactions to this component of the shot, including meningitis, febrile convulsions, encephalitis, and epilepsy.[29]

According to Wellcome, the rubella portion of the vaccine causes arthritis in 3 percent of child vaccinees and 12 to 20 percent of adult women recipients. "Symptoms may persist for a matter of months or, on rare occasions, for years," the company reports; effects range from mild aches in the joints to extreme crippling.[30]

Robert Mendelsohn, MD, in reporting on the work of Aubrey Tingle, MD—a pediatric immunologist at Children's Hospital in Vancouver, British Columbia—points out that 30 percent of adults exposed to rubella vaccine developed arthritis two to four weeks afterward. Tingle also found the rubella virus in one-third of all adults and children with rheumatoid arthritis.[31]

This jibes with a 1970 Department of Health, Education and Welfare report citing that as many as "26 percent of children receiving rubella vaccination in national testing programs developed arthralgia and arthritis. Many had to seek medical attention, and some were hospitalized to test for rheumatic fever and rheumatoid arthritis."[32]

Morris testified against these and other vaccines in congressional hearings and, in the process, paved the way for the National Childhood Vaccine Injury Act that now awards remuneration to victims of vaccines. In his view, all statistics thus far published on side effects of the triple jab are extremely conservative. "We only hear about the encephalitis and the deaths," he says. "But there is an entire spectrum of reactions between fever and death, and it's all those things in between that never get reported."[33]

Part of that spectrum involves the temporary or imperfect immunity conferred by the vaccine. Many vaccinated children, for example, may grow up susceptible to measles, mumps, or rubella—each of which is far more serious, even deadly, in adulthood. Ample evidence already indicates that vaccinated children can contract new diseases such as atypical measles, which is more serious than the ordinary variety, often causing pneumonia and severe pain.[34]

Of special concern is the high failure rate of the rubella portion of the shot—sometimes within only five years of vaccination. This part of the vaccine was designed to eliminate German measles not so much in young children as among women of childbearing age. The hope was to counteract the likelihood of contracting the disease while pregnant and thus bearing a child with possible birth defects. The vaccine, however, wears off; when it does, one becomes susceptible to German measles. *In fact, vaccinated populations of women are more likely to contract the illness during pregnancy than are those who had German measles naturally in childhood, because the illness itself tends to confer lifelong immunity.*

TOWARD TRUE IMMUNITY

How I would love to get my hands on a magic bullet that would wipe out in an instant all the feverish, sleepless nights my little one may have to suffer as she struggles through the various childhood illnesses—for the battle, I've decided, is the best option there is. The vaccine presently on offer is simply too experimental, too ineffective, and too risky; and the illnesses it is designed to prevent are rarely life threatening to healthy, well-nourished children, especially those who've been breastfed.

Even when the most serious of these illnesses strikes, less drastic health measures are available. *The Lancet* recently reported that giving vitamin A to children with severe measles lessens the complications of illness and the chances of dying. Indeed, author Gerald T. Keusch, MD, of Boston's New England Medical Center, concluded that children benefit from appropriate doses of vitamin A whenever they exhibit a vitamin A deficiency or even the possibility of complications due to measles.[35]

Two of Caitlin's unvaccinated friends recently came down with measles. Their reactions were mild, a bit like the flu. Now they will have true immunity to measles for the rest of their lives. I am putting my money where their mothers put theirs: on nature's own tried-and-tested immunization program.

NOTES

1. "Measles: United States, 1990," *Journal of the American Medical Association* (26 June 1991): 3227.

2. William K. Stevens, "Despite Vaccine, Perilous Measles Won't Go Away," *The New York Times* (14 March 1989): C–6.

3. "Measles Immunization: Recommendations, Challenges and More Information" (editorial), *Journal of the American Medical Association* (24 April 1991): 2111.

4. "Secretary of Health, Human Services to Hear Recommendations for Improving Immunization," *Journal of the American Medical Association* (17 October 1990): 1925.

5. "Campus Ills," *Time* Magazine (11 March 1985): 66.

6. "Measles Prevention: Supplementary Statement," *Journal of the American Medical Association* (10 February 1989): 827.

7. Tracy L. Gustafson et al., "Measles Outbreak in a Fully Immunized Secondary School Population," *New England Journal of Medicine* (26 March 1987): 771–774.

8. "Measles in the USA," *The Pediatric Infectious Disease Journal Newsletter* (September 1987): 18.

9. *Morbidity and Mortality Weekly Report* (6 June 1987); cited in Robert S. Mendelsohn, *But Doctor . . . About That Shot* (Chicago, IL: The People's Doctor, 1988), 81.

10. Laurie E. Markowitz et al., "Patterns of Transmission in Measles Outbreaks in the United States: 1985–6," *New England Journal of Medicine* (12 January 1989): 75.

11. See Note 9, 21.

12. M. G. Cusi et al. (correspondence), *The Lancet* (27 October 1990): 1070.

13. David Isaacs and Margaret Menser, "Modern Vaccines: Measles, Mumps, Rubella, and Varicella," *The Lancet* (27 October 1990): 1385.

14. J. T. Jabbour et al., "Epidemiology of Subacute Sclerosing Panencephalitis (SSPE)," *Journal of the American Medical Association* (15 May 1972): 959.

15. Neal A. Halsey et al., "Risk Factors in Subacute Sclerosing Panencephalitis: A Case Control Study," *Journal of the American Medical Association* (4 November 1980): 415–424.

16. New York Times News Service.

17. Dr. Norman Begg, in an interview with the author (December 1989).

18. Ibid.

19. See Note 13, 1385.

20. H. Allerdist, "Neurological Complications Following Measles Vaccination"; presented at the International Symposium on Immunization: Benefit versus Risk Factors, in Brussels (1978); published in *Development of Biological Standards* 432 (1979): 259–264.

21. Dr. J. Anthony Morris, in an interview with the author (December 1989).

22. "Mumps, Meningitis and MMR Vaccination" (editorial), *The Lancet* (28 October 1989): 1016.

23. *ABPI Data Sheet Compendium, 1989–90* (London, England: Datapharm Publications, 1989), 1717.

24. See Note 15, 417–421.

25. Jane McDonald et al., "Clinical and Epidemiological Features of Mumps Meningoencephalitis and Possible Vaccine-Related Disease," *Pediatric Infectious Disease Journal* (November 1989): 751–754.

26. See Note 22, 1017.

27. Milan Cizman et al., "Aseptic Meningitis after Vaccination against Measles and Mumps," *Pediatric Infectious Disease Journal* (May 1989): 302.

28. James A. Gray and Sheila M. Burns (correspondence), *The Lancet* (14 October 1989): 98.

29. W. Ehrengut (correspondence), *The Lancet* (23 September 1989): 751.

30. See Note 23, 1718.

31. See Note 9, 30.

32. *Science* (26 March 1977); cited in Walene James, *Immunization: The Reality behind the Myth* (Hadley, MA: Bergin & Garvey, 1988), 12.

33. Dr. J. Anthony Morris, in an interview with the author (January 1990).

34. Z. Spirer et al. (correspondence), *Pediatric Infectious Disease Journal* (March 1986): 276–277.

35. Gerald T. Keusch, "Vitamin A Supplements—Too Good Not to Be True," *New England Journal of Medicine* (4 October 1990): 985–987.

THE CHICKENPOX VACCINE
BY MARYANN NAPOLI

Maryann Napoli is cofounder and associate director of the Center for Medical Consumers and editor of HealthFacts *newsletter. She and her husband, Richard, have been married more than 30 years and have two daughters, both of whom work in the women's health movement.*

The chickenpox vaccine is now available, despite doubts raised by some experts about the merits of mass immunization for a relatively minor childhood illness. The vaccine was developed more than 13 years ago to protect high-risk children, such as those with AIDS and leukemia, from severe, potentially fatal complications. But a continuing controversy over its necessity for healthy children delayed the vaccine's approval.

In March 1995, the FDA approved the licensure of a live attenuated varicella (chickenpox) vaccine. Wide acceptance was guaranteed when, in May 1995, the American Academy of Pediatrics announced that it should be given to all children, ages one to 18 years old, who haven't had chickenpox.

Opponents of universal immunization are concerned about the long-term safety and effectiveness of the vaccine. Proponents insist that chickenpox is not always a minor illness, accounting for 56 deaths in otherwise healthy children and more than 9,900 hospitalizations annually. But a physician at the Centers for Disease Control and Prevention, who preferred to remain anonymous, said in a telephone interview that the varicella-related deaths and complications were not the main consideration for the development of the new vaccine. Rather, it was driven by economic considerations that took into account the number of workdays lost by parents who had to stay home with a sick child.

The most serious concern raised by the consumer-led National Vaccine Information Center is the unknown long-term effects. (No studies of children given the chickenpox vaccine have followed participants longer than ten years.) "That's an understandable concern, and one that is raised with the introduction of almost all new childhood vaccines and shown to be incorrect," said Neal Halsey, MD, of the American Academy of Pediatrics committee on infectious disease.

He continued, "The end result has been a marked protection against the diseases of children, and subsequently, of adults. You can't expect to have 20 years of follow-up on something that's brand new. This is true of any other new drug or new surgical procedure. With most new vaccines, the children have been followed for only about three or four years."

The debate over the chickenpox vaccine's usefulness for healthy children made the front page of the *New York Times* three years ago. "Do you want to give a vaccine with unknown side effects—to prevent a very mild disease?" asked Phillip Brunnell, head of pediatric infectious disease at Cedars Sinai Hospital in Los Angeles in the 1993 *Times* interview. "If parents' lost work is the problem, then maybe we should send the children back to school sooner," he said, noting that many schools won't permit the child to return before the lesions disappear completely, though most feel well enough far earlier. Ironically, the disease is most contagious *before* the rash appears. Brunnell and other experts were quoted in the article as agreeing with this statement: "To justify vaccinating everyone against a disease that for most is more inconvenient than harmful, the shot itself must be unquestionably safe."

Today, Brunnell has changed his mind. "Now that it's licensed, I think everyone should be vaccinated," he said in a recent phone interview. "To have a partially immunized population is bad because it would increase the likelihood of susceptible adults who would get the disease when it's more severe." He conceded that the unknown long-term effects are a concern. For example, there is a question of whether this live, though weakened, strain of the varicella-zoster virus is more likely to be reactivated later in life and cause the painful rash known as shingles.

The National Vaccination Information Center contends that this is yet another example of an immunization that could backfire. The vaccine may be effective only for a limited time, perhaps ten years, which could have the effect of shifting chickenpox to the adult population, among whom it poses serious risks, such as pneumonia and inflammation of the brain.

This has already occurred in some people given the measles vaccine. Before this vaccine was introduced in 1957, virtually everyone got measles in childhood; the disease rarely occurred in adults and infants under age one, when serious complications are more likely.

Although the measles vaccine was supposed to have wiped out

measles, an outbreak began in 1989. In 1990 alone, there were 90 deaths from measles. Low immunization rates in some inner-city populations were widely cited as the cause, but 40 percent of the cases occurred in appropriately vaccinated children. The largest increase in measles incidence took place in adults over 25 years of age and in infants under the age of one. According to the National Vaccine Information Center, the increase in measles among infants was due to the fact that their vaccinated mothers were unable to pass on protective antibodies.

Barbara Loe Fisher, the National Vaccine Information Center's president and cofounder, is concerned about the chickenpox vaccine's implications for the immune system. "By advocating this vaccine for everyone, not just high-risk children, they are putting older children and adults at risk, and there will no longer be as much chickenpox in the child population. Therefore, the opportunity to have permanent immunity is lost," she said.

The varicella vaccine is 70 to 90 percent effective. Whether there will be a need for a booster shot is unclear, but many believe it is likely. Furthermore, some pediatricians have raised the question of how many immunizations a baby can be given safely. Many pediatricians rebelled after the last vaccine recommendation (for hepatitis B) and refused to comply. Currently, babies receive multiple vaccinations for nine diseases.

CONSIDERING VARICELLA
BY ANNE MONTGOMERY

The new varicella vaccine is now being recommended by major groups for all children, to be given at the same time as the MMR. A combination MMR-varicella vaccine will probably be available sometime. I believe the varicella vaccine has an important role to play, but I am skeptical about this universal recommendation. I am afraid that we will see similarities to measles: Young children won't get the disease and won't develop lifelong protection from the virus. We will see outbreaks in young adults, in whom the disease can be very serious, and in pregnant women, who will become ill and who could infect their newborns—with serious results. I hope we have learned from measles and will have an appropriate booster program in place before such outbreaks occur. It is also somewhat reassuring that we have effective passive immunity (Varicella-Zoster Immune Globulin, or V-ZIG) and antiviral medications available to deal with these situations.

The societal cost-benefit analysis of the vaccine included the very large dollar cost of parental work time lost. This benefit does not apply to people who are caring for their children at home. People using small daycares with healthy children also often decide that children can return after they are no longer sick but before they are completely healed, since they were more infectious the day before they got the first spots than they are when healing. I am also philosophically uncomfortable with a society that does not support parents' staying home with sick children.

The most prudent recommendation I have seen regarding varicella immunization is to immunize anyone who gets to be about 11 without having chickenpox. This will prevent the majority of the serious cases of chickenpox and will also be cost-effective, since a single dose is needed up until ages 11 to 12; children over 13 require two doses of vaccine. There should be enough disease still around for most young children to have chickenpox and develop lifelong immunity from natural disease. While I will give varicella vaccine to a young child whose parents request it, I am currently recommending this approach when asked for my advice. Chickenpox can be a miserable and sometimes disfiguring disease even for young children, so I may be swayed toward earlier vaccination, particularly once the vaccine develops a long-term track record. For now, though, I remain cautious about it.

CHICKENPOX: LIVE AND LET LIVE?
BY JAY GORDON

The chickenpox vaccine is finally here. I still think that getting the natural disease is better, but I'm afraid that may not be possible as the Varivax shot puts a halt to all those lovely chickenpox epidemics that used to sweep through school, canceling Christmas or Thanksgiving vacations in their wake. Any child over age one can receive this shot, but I'd prefer to give it primarily to older children who have already had a chance to get the disease and haven't, and thus may be at a much higher risk of contracting a severe case. All adults without chickenpox immunity should strongly consider getting this vaccine. I am very willing to use the vaccine because I think it's safe. Children need one dose, and teenagers and adults need two. Zovirax will lessen a case of chickenpox if given in the first 24 to 48 hours but is not recommended for routine childhood cases.

Pertussis (Whooping Cough)
By Carol Miller

Pertussis is an infectious disease of childhood, associated with a specific bacteria. It can sometimes have dramatic and alarming symptoms. Usually it is characterized by a period of cold symptoms followed by an extended period (four to six weeks) of violent coughing. The disease primarily occurs in infants and young children. Deaths from whooping cough are usually due to complicating respiratory infection. Pneumonia is responsible for 90 percent of these deaths in children under three years of age.

In the past ten years 0.4 percent of pertussis cases have proved fatal. The incidence of the disease has steadily decreased in the last 40 years. There were 21,334 cases reported in California in 1941 and only 147 reported in 1980.

Immunity

Little or no immunity is transferred from the mother to the newborn infant. Active immunization with pertussis vaccine is claimed to prevent the disease or lessen the severity of the attack. An attack of the actual disease does not necessarily confer permanent immunity.

Efficacy

The natural history of this disease shows a great reduction in mortality in England long before the vaccine was introduced. Mortality rates continued to decline after the introduction of immunization, but the rate of decline was not significantly greater than before.

Immunization with pertussis vaccine is claimed to induce protective levels of immunity in about 75 percent of those vaccinated. A recent carefully designed but theoretical analysis of pertussis and immunization predicted that the incidence of pertussis would increase 71 times a few years after the cessation of immunizations.

There is conflicting evidence, however, from recent outbreaks of the illness. In one recent report of 8,092 cases of whooping cough, 1,940 (24 percent) were fully immunized and only 2,424 (30 percent) were definitely not immunized. Among 85 fully immunized children studied during an epidemic in 1978, at least 46 developed whooping cough.

SAFETY

Immunization with pertussis vaccine has been clearly shown to cause a significant number of adverse reactions, some very serious. The most frequent include fevers, behavioral changes (including crying, irritability, and a peculiar screaming syndrome), and redness, swelling, and tenderness at the injection site.

More serious reactions include encephalitis, convulsions, and brain damage, leading in a sizable number of cases to persistent disease or death. No one is sure how frequently these serious reactions occur; estimates range from one in 3,600 to one in 500,000. During 1969 to 1974 in Great Britain, when 64 deaths from whooping cough were reported, there were 56 cases of brain damage following vaccination. In this country, 46 deaths after DPT (diphtheria-pertussis-tetanus) vaccination were reported in 1979, 33 of them sudden infant deaths. (The pertussis component of the DPT immunization is thought to be responsible for serious reactions following the injection.) It is not clear whether these deaths were caused by the immunization.

In spite of these dangers, the American Academy of Pediatrics has concluded that the benefits of pertussis immunization outweigh the risks. Advocates of immunization say that the risk of convulsions and brain damage following whooping cough is greater than that following vaccination. They also point to a recent significant increase in whooping cough in Great Britain paralleling the decline of immunization as evidence of the necessity for immunization. There is sharp controversy, however, about the reasons for this spread of the disease.

DIAGNOSIS

The characteristic cough of pertussis makes the disease easy to diagnose. The cough comes in paroxysms and is often preceded by a feeling of apprehension or anxiety and tightness in the chest. The cough itself consists of short, explosive expirations in rapid succession followed by a long, crowing inspiration. During the coughing the child's face may become red or even blue, the eyes bulge, and the tongue protrudes. A number of such paroxysms are sometimes followed by spitting up a mucus plug and vomiting. This will end the attack, and the child will rest or appear dazed. Many of these attacks may occur in one day, more frequently at night and in a stuffy room.

They may be brought on by physical exertion, crying, and often by eating and drinking. Attacks diminish when the child is concentrating on toys, books, and so forth. Infants, however, do not always have "whooping" with their coughing.

Diagnosis is assisted by identifying the organism (*B. pertussis*) during the first one or two weeks of illness. After that it becomes difficult to culture the bacteria. High white blood cell counts (20,000 per cu. mm) with a predominance of lymphocytes (60 percent) are characteristic. Complications of pertussis may include cerebral hemorrhage, convulsions, and brain damage, as well as pneumonia, emphysema, or collapsed lung.

TREATMENT

Standard treatment with antibiotics may help reduce the period of contagion to others and prevent complications. Pertussis immune globula may help shorten the illness and prevent complications and deaths in children under two. Good intensive nursing care is essential.

SUMMARY

Pertussis vaccine is questionably effective and can cause serious side effects in a small number of people. Whooping cough can be a severe illness, and has in the past resulted in many deaths, though the percentage of fatalities is now very low. The ultimate decision and responsibility for immunizing against pertussis must rest with the child's parents. In general, the clinic does not recommend the administration of this vaccination.

Excerpted with permission from an out-of-print booklet, Immunizations: Are They Necessary? *by Carol Miller, a past publication of the Hering Family Health Clinic, Berkeley, California.*

VACCINATIONS
BY MAGDA KRANCE

Risks and rates of diseases, risks and rates of side effects of recommended vaccinations. (Courtesy of Centers for Disease Control, Atlanta; data current as of 1991)

DIPHTHERIA
1 case reported in United States in 1988

Can cause infection in nose, throat, and skin; can interfere with breathing; sometimes causes heart failure or paralysis. 1:10 die from it in the United States.

PERTUSSIS
3,008 cases reported in United States in 1988

Also called whooping cough; causes severe coughing spells that can interfere with eating, drinking, and breathing. In the United States, 70 percent of reported cases occur in children under five years of age; more than 50 percent of those under one year of age are hospitalized. In the United States, 1:4 children with pertussis develop pneumonia. 22:1,000 develop convulsions and/or other brain problems. An average of nine deaths a year are caused by pertussis in the United States.

TETANUS
49 cases reported in United States in 1988

Also called lockjaw; results when wounds are infected with tetanus bacteria, which are often found in dirt. If the wound is not properly cleaned, a poison forms in the wound and causes muscle spasms. In the United States, 4:10 who get tetanus die from it.

MUMPS
4,730 cases reported in United States in 1988

Usually produces fever, headache, and inflammation of salivary glands, causing cheeks to swell. Can be more serious, resulting in mild meningitis in 1:10 children. More rarely, can cause deafness or encephalitis. In adolescent or adult males who get mumps, 1:4 can develop painful inflammation of the testicles, causing sterility in rare cases.

RUBELLA

221 cases reported in United States in 1988

Also called German measles. Usually very mild, causing slight fever, rash, and swelling of neck glands. Lasts about three days. In adult women, may cause joint swelling for one to two weeks. Very rarely, can cause encephalitis or purpura (temporary bleeding disorder). In pregnant women, can cause miscarriage or birth defects.

POLIO

2 cases reported in United States in 1988

Virus disease that can cause permanent crippling and occasionally death.

MEASLES

3,643 cases reported in United States in 1988

Usually causes rash, high fever, cough, runny nose, watery eyes for one to two weeks. Can be more serious: causes ear infection or pneumonia in 1:10 children who get it; causes encephalitis in 1:1,000 children who get it, which can lead to convulsions, deafness, or mental retardation. 2:10,000 children who contract measles die from it. *

*According to George Seastrom of the CDC's Immunizations Division, as of June 25, 1989, there was a 370 percent increase in measles cases over the 1988 total. As of that date there were 7,022 cases of measles reported, as opposed to 1,492 cases reported the previous year at the same time.

According to Seastrom, "Of school-age children, over 90 percent have been adequately vaccinated. As far as preschoolers are concerned, depending on the area of the country, it would range from 40 to 60 percent." The percentages reflect the fact that some parents may not take their children in for inoculation until they are required to do so, when the children are ready to enter school. (Many daycare centers and preschools also require proof of immunizations before admitting children.) According to Samuel Katz of Duke University's School of Medicine, there is a drop in the numbers of children being immunized, because their parents were not yet born during the prevaccine epidemics and are thus unaware of the dangers.

VACCINES—RATE OF PROTECTION, SIDE EFFECTS, RATE OF OCCURRENCE, AND CONTRAINDICATIONS

DPT/DT/TD (DIPHTHERIA-PERTUSSIS-TETANUS)

More than 95 percent of those who receive the full series of shots are protected from tetanus. Diphtheria and pertussis parts of the vaccine are not as effective, but still protect most children from getting the disease and make the disease milder for those who do get it.

With DPT vaccine, most children will have a slight fever and be irritable within two days of inoculation. Half will have some soreness and swelling in the shot area. In 1:330 shots, a temperature of 105° or more may occur. In 1:100 shots, continuous crying for three or more hours may result. In 1:900 shots, unusual high-pitched crying may occur. In 1:1,750 cases, convulsions, limpness, or paleness may be caused by the shot. In 1:10,000 shots, severe brain problems may occur, and in 1:310,000 shots, permanent brain damage may result. These side effects are caused by the pertussis component of the shot; DT or TD shots may cause soreness and slight fever.

Children who have had a serious reaction to a DPT shot should not receive additional pertussis vaccine. Children who have previously had a convulsion or are suspected of having any nervous system problem should not receive DPT vaccine without thorough medical evaluation; likewise if there is any family history of convulsions or nervous system problems. Children who are currently sick should not receive DPT until they are well. And children undergoing treatment that may lower resistance to infection (e.g., cortisone, prednisone, radiation therapy, and so forth) should not receive DPT.

MMR (MEASLES, MUMPS, RUBELLA)

About 90 percent of those who are inoculated will have protection, probably for life, if not vaccinated before the age of 15 months. 1:5 children will get a rash or slight fever lasting a few days one to two weeks after receiving the measles vaccine. Occasionally, there may be mild swelling of salivary glands caused by the mumps vaccine. 1:7 children will get a rash or some swelling of neck glands one or two weeks after getting rubella vaccine. 1:20 children will have some aching or swelling of joints one to three weeks after receiving rubella vaccine, lasting a few days. In adults, 4:10 may have temporary joint swelling after rubella vaccine; 2:100 may develop true arthritis after the vaccine. Very rarely, children may develop encephalitis, convulsions with fever, and neurological problems after the MMR vaccinations.

Anyone who is currently sick should not have the MMR shot until healthy. Anyone who has had a severe allergic reaction to eating eggs should not take the measles or mumps components. Anyone with cancer, leukemia, or lymphoma should not take the shot, nor should anyone taking medication that reduces resistance to infection.

OPV (ORAL POLIO VACCINE)

In more than 90 percent of those inoculated, OPV gives long-term, possibly lifelong protection. 1:8,100,000 doses of OPV causes paralytic polio in the person vaccinated. 1:5,000,000 doses may cause paralytic polio in a close contact of a recently vaccinated person.

OPV should not be taken by anyone with cancer, leukemia, or lymphoma; by anyone taking medication that reduces resistance to infection; by anyone living in the same household with anyone who has any of the above conditions; by anyone who is currently sick; or by pregnant women. Anyone over the age of 18 should avoid inoculation unless there is an outbreak in the community.

IPV (INJECTABLE POLIO VACCINE)

Also called killed polio vaccine; it has no known risk of causing paralytic polio. IPV is recommended for persons with low resistance to serious infections, or for those living with persons with low resistance. It may also be recommended for previously unvaccinated adults whose children are to be vaccinated with OPV.

INFORMED CONSENT

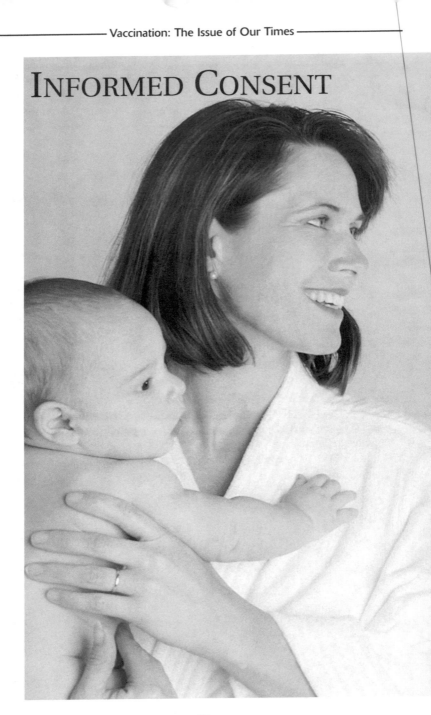

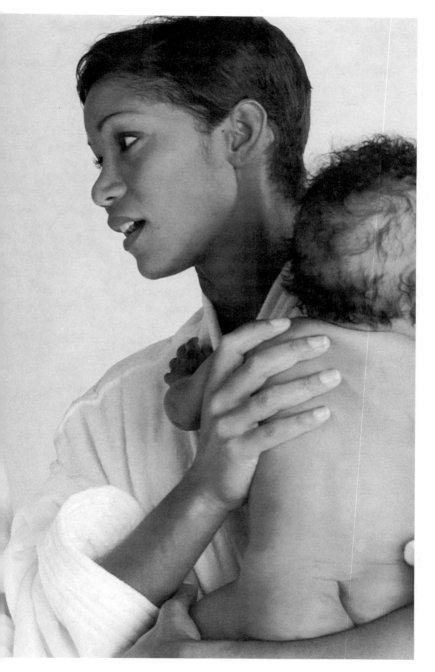

VACCINE POLICY: A SHOT AT YOUR RIGHTS?

BY PEGGIE CYPHER

Peggie Cypher is a writer and educator. She lives in the Midwest with her husband, Paul, and their son, Neil (4).

More than 37,000 reports of adverse reactions to vaccines, including 471 deaths, were reported by the Food and Drug Administration's Vaccine Adverse Events Reporting System between July 1990 and March 1994. This number may be even greater, as some adverse reactions are never reported. In the past, parents have had the right to seek compensation for their children who have been injured by vaccines and to take a legal exemption not to immunize their children at all. But a series of actions by federal and state governments has threatened those rights. Here's what's happening and what you can do.

PHILOSOPHICAL EXEMPTIONS

Until recently, 19 states granted the right of parents to seek philosophical exemptions—the option to decline immunizations for personal and philosophical reasons—but in the push to have children 100 percent vaccinated by the year 2000, some states, backed by their departments of health, have abolished them.

In Michigan, State Representative Lyn Bankes has introduced legislation to do away with the philosophical exemption. [1] The bill, which is expected to enter committee this year, is being opposed by a group called Michigan Opposing Mandatory Vaccines (MOM). "Parents should have the right to make healthcare decisions for their children and themselves," says Suzanne Lewandowski, chairperson of MOM.

Dr. Kristine Severyn, registered pharmacist and director of Ohio Parents for Vaccine Safety (OPVS) agrees. Informed consent is a basic tenet of medicine. It implies voluntary consent. Parents have the choice not to fill prescriptions—they can talk to doctors about non-drug therapy. But with mandatory vaccination laws for school and daycare and college admission, that class of medicine is put in a different legal category." According to Severyn, most developed countries, including Canada, Japan, and those in Western Europe, have philosophical exemptions.

The fight for philosophical exemption in Texas is an uphill battle, but imperative given the fact that more and more vaccines are being required by state governments, say Karin Schumacher, president of Vaccine Information Awareness in Texas. Texas recently mandated the hepatitis B vaccine for all school-age children. Hepatitis B is a disease usually found among intravenous drug users and the sexually promiscuous. "The vaccine issue goes to the core of our freedom, which is what America is about," say Schumacher. "We must have the freedom to choose and then respect everyone's choice."

Vaccine Tracking Systems

A key component of the Childhood Immunization Act of 1992 was the creation of a national vaccination tracking system that would link a person's vaccination status to his or her birth certificate and Social Security number. Though the tracking system was cut by Congress in an effort not to increase the deficit, 19 states, including Mississippi, Connecticut, Texas, and New York, are already establishing registries to monitor the immunization status of children.

Public Assistance and Vaccinations

The trend of states to link public assistance and tax-supported healthcare plans to mandatory vaccinations also denies a large number of people informed consent. Effective last summer, applicants to Aid to Families with Dependent Children (AFDC) in Indiana had to sign a "Personal Responsibility Agreement," which obligates them to have their children vaccinated. Failure to have children immunized on schedule results in the loss of $90 per month in public assistance. Texas is working toward a similar provision, where recipients of AFDC will lose $25 per month per child unless they show proof of immunization. Maryland and Georgia have also made public assistance contingent on having children vaccinated.

Under Tennessee's health plan for state employees and poor people (TennCare), healthcare practitioners are not paid in full if all the children on the physician's patient list are not vaccinated. [2]A similar plan is being proposed for OhioCare, where payments would be withheld from HMOs for not vaccinating a designated percentage of their patient populations. Dr. Severyn of Ohio Parents for Vaccine Safety worries that if states are successful in linking vaccinations to tax-supported medical care, the government may one day force private health insurance companies to require families to immunize their children or face loss of benefits.

VACCINE COMPENSATION PROGRAM

The National Childhood Vaccine Injury Act was created by Congress in 1986 to allow parents to seek compensation for children adversely affected by vaccines. But in February 1995, under the direction of Health and Human Services Secretary Donna Shalala, the act was revised to more narrowly define what constitutes vaccine injury. The adverse reactions now associated with a DPT shot, for example, are anaphylaxis occurring within four hours (reduced from 24 in the old injury table) and encephalopathy (brain inflammation) occurring within 72 hours. Under the new definition of encephalopathy, children would have to show a "significantly decreased level of consciousness" for more than 24 hours or be hospitalized in order to qualify. Babies exhibiting symptoms such as high-pitched screaming, shock collapse, and residue seizure disorder—symptoms that may lead to permanent neurological damage—may no longer be presumed eligible for compensation. [3]Over $500 million has been paid out in compensation since 1990, with the majority of cases citing these classic symptoms, says Kathi Williams, director of the National Vaccine Information Center and Dissatisfied Parents Together (NVIC/DPT).

A recent Supreme Court ruling in Indiana has also made it more difficult for parents whose children were injured by vaccines to seek compensation. The parents of Maggie Whitecotton won compensation in 1994 from a federal appeals court for their daughter's injury after a DPT shot. But the ruling was recently overturned by the Supreme Court, which stated that proof is required that children had no symptoms of a particular injury prior to vaccination.[4]

When states make vaccinations law, and drug manufacturers take none of the risk for adverse reactions, Severyn believes there is no incentive for companies to make safer products. "The parents are left holding the bag."

The National Childhood Vaccine Injury Act was created as a nonadversarial alternative to lawsuits against drug companies and physicians. NVIC/DPT urges parents concerned with this compensation program to register their views at the opinion line at the White House (202-456-1111) or by fax (202-456-2461). You can also call your congressional representative (202-224-3121) or write to Donna Shalala at 200 Independence Avenue, Room 615F, Washington, DC 20202, fax (202-690-7203).

NOTES

1. R. Mishra, "Lawmakers' Plan Seeks to Scale Back Vaccine Exemptions," *Detroit Free Press* (31 May 1995).

2. J. Woo and W. Lambert, "Refusal to Immunize Youngster Said to Violate Child-Neglect Laws," *Wall Street Journal* (22 February 1993).

3. *Federal Register* 60 (8 February 1995).

4. Associated Press (wire), "Top Court Toughens Vaccination Injury Rule" (12 April 1995).

ADVERSE EFFECTS OF CHILDHOOD VACCINES
BY THE INSTITUTE OF MEDICINE

EVIDENCE ESTABLISHES A CAUSAL RELATION BETWEEN
THE FOLLOWING:

Diphtheria and Tetanus Toxoids	Anaphylaxis
Measles Vaccine	Death from measles-strain viral infection
MMR Vaccine	Thrombocytopenia Anaphylaxis
Oral Polio Vaccine (OPV)	Poliomyelitis in recipient or contact
	Death from polio vaccine-strain viral infection
Hepatitis B Vaccine	Anaphylaxis

EVIDENCE INDICATES A CAUSAL RELATION BETWEEN
THE FOLLOWING:

DPT Vaccine	Anaphylaxis
	Protracted, inconsolable crying
Rubella Vaccine	Acute arthritis

EVIDENCE IS CONSISTENT WITH A CAUSAL RELATION
BETWEEN THE FOLLOWING:

DPT Vaccine	Acute encephalopathy Shock Unusual "shock-like state"
Rubella Vaccine	Chronic arthritis

EVIDENCE FAVORS ACCEPTANCE OF A CAUSAL RELATION BETWEEN THE FOLLOWING:

Diphtheria and Tetanus Toxoids	Guillain-Barré syndrome Brachial neuritis
Measles Vaccine	Anaphylaxis
OPV/IPVb Vaccine	Guillain-Barré syndrome
H. influenzae type b	Early-onset *H. influenzae* b disease in 18 months or older who receive first vaccine with unconjugated PRP vaccine

SOURCES

Howson, Christopher P., et al. *Adverse Effects of Pertussis and Rubella Vaccines: A Report of the Committee to Review the Adverse Consequences of Pertussis and Rubella Vaccines*, Division of Health Promotion and Disease Prevention, Institute of Medicine. Washington, DC: National Academy Press, 1991.

Stratton, Kathleen, et al. *Adverse Events Associated with Childhood Vaccines: Evidence Bearing on Causality*, Vaccine Safety Committee, Division of Health Promotion and Disease Prevention, Institute of Medicine. Washington, DC: National Academy Press, 1994.

Adverse Effects of Pertussis and Rubella Vaccines (1991) and *Adverse Events Associated with Childhood Vaccines* (1994) are two reports researched by the Institute of Medicine and published by the National Academy Press. The reports are the work of a project approved by the Governing Board of the National Research Council, whose members are drawn from the councils of the National Academy of Sciences, the National Academy of Engineering, and the Institute of Medicine. Committee members responsible for the report were chosen for special competencies and with regard for appropriate balance.

The Institute of Medicine was chartered in 1970 by the National Academy of Sciences to enlist distinguished members of the appropriate professions in the examination of policy matters pertaining to the health of the public. In this, the institute acts, under the academy's 1863 congressional charter responsibility, to be an adviser to the federal government and act upon its own initiative to identify issues of medical care, research, and education.

For the vast majority of vaccine-adverse event relations studied, the data came predominantly from uncontrolled studies and case reports. Most of the pathologic conditions studied are rare in the general population. The risk of developing these conditions because of vaccination would seem to be low.

NEED FOR RESEARCH AND SURVEILLANCE

During its attempt to find evidence regarding causality, the committee identified needs for research and surveillance of adverse events. Work in these areas will help to ensure that all vaccines used are as free from the risk of causing adverse events as possible. Some of the needs identified are for increased surveillance of reports of demylinating disease and arthritis following hepatitis B vaccinations, better follow-up reports of death and other serious adverse events following vaccinations, increased use of large databases (currently used only on a small scale) to supplement passive surveillance reporting systems, and disease registries for the rare pathologic conditions studied by the committee.

Excerpted with permission from Adverse Effects of Pertussis and Rubella Vaccines *and* Adverse Events Associated with Childhood Vaccines, *National Academy Press, 1991 and 1994.*

VACCINATION PRECAUTIONS
BY VICKI GILES

"Vaccinations and Individual Freedom" first appeared in
Mothering, *no. 39 (Spring 1986).*

There can be no doubt that any medicine that is potent enough to be effective has at least some potential for toxicity as well. Parents should be aware of the following precautions when dealing with routine vaccinations:

Do not allow your child to be immunized if he or she has been ill or has had a cold or runny nose within the last 48 hours. Vaccinations provide immunity by going directly into the bloodstream, and an immune system that is already taxed is more likely to react badly to immunization. Vaccinations also affect the lymphatic system, which may already be stressed by a cold or runny nose.

If you wish to have your child vaccinated, consider beginning at six months rather than six weeks. If your child was small for gestational age or was born prematurely, consider waiting even longer. Although most physicians would recommend that immunizations be started at six weeks because the risk of pertussis, for example, is greater in infancy, there have never been any controlled studies done to determine whether or not an infant under six months of age can actually build immunity when immunized. Booster shots became popular to protect against the possibility that early immunity may not develop through immunization.

In Great Britain, vaccinations are started at six months of age. Why do we start them so much sooner in the US? The major reasoning for beginning vaccinations so early comes from a study conducted by Parke-Davis in 1962, which concluded that it is more likely that children will receive the entire series of vaccinations if they are begun early in infancy. And since most babies visit the doctor at four to six weeks for a checkup, it is more convenient for the health practitioner to start the series of immunizations at this time.

If you have a family history of central nervous system disease, deafness, blindness, convulsions, or life-threatening allergies, the pertussis vaccine may be contraindicated for your child. The pertussis part of the diphtheria-pertussis-tetanus (DPT) vaccine is considered quite crude. The "whole-cell" pertussis vaccine given to US children has not been separated; the child receives the part of the pertussis cell that generates immunity to the disease along with the part that causes toxic reactions. Current research may be able to isolate the toxic element.

If one child in your family has had a serious reaction to the pertussis vaccine, the child's siblings should probably not receive the vaccine. Children in the same family tend to react similarly to the pertussis vaccine. The reason for this is not clear.

If your child has exhibited a severe reaction to the pertussis vaccine, immediately find a physician who will verify the reaction and write in your child's permanent medical record that he or she should never again receive a pertussis shot. Once a particular child has reacted seriously, additional doses will frequently cause more serious reactions. A serious reaction to vaccination may include any of the following: excessive, high-pitched screaming (the high-pitched scream is suggestive of central nervous system irritation); severe swelling or redness at the site of the injection; fever lasting several days; collapse or extreme lethargy; grayish skin color and cool extremities; or convulsions.

If your child exhibits any of these symptoms, be sure to notify your health professionals and urge them to report the reaction to the federal Centers for Disease Control (CDC) in Atlanta, along with the lot and batch number of the vaccination given. Some physicians might not consider local swelling and fever lasting several days to be severe reactions, but there have been cases of children who have exhibited swelling and fever reactions to a first immunization and more severe reactions to a second one, so even swelling and fever should not be discounted.

Some practitioners suggest a half dose followed by another half dose for children who have exhibited a toxic reaction to the vaccine. However, all available evidence indicates that giving the child a half dose of DPT, followed one week later by another half dose, does *not* lessen the potential for toxic reaction.

Always write down the batch and lot number of any vaccine that your child is given. Be sure to look carefully at the vial whenever your child is given a vaccination. It is possible for a person to make a mistake and give your child the wrong vaccine.

If for any reason your child becomes ill enough to be hospitalized within two weeks following a vaccination, fully describe the course of illness to the health center where the child was given the vaccination. Urge the healthcare professionals to report the reaction, batch, and lot number to the CDC. This will help the CDC statistically analyze whether the batch is particularly reactive or whether your child is overly sensitive to vaccination.

Many, perhaps most, doctors do not consistently report adverse reactions to vaccines. Consequently, the CDC lacks clinical figures for how often a particular vaccine is reactive.

For about two weeks after receiving the "live" polio vaccine, keep your child away from anyone who is not fully immunized against polio and anyone who has an immune deficiency (for example, acquired immune deficiency syndrome or a deficiency due to chemotherapy) for that person's own protection. The "live" polio vaccine, a live virus, is contagious. Because the disease is carried in the bodily excretions, it is especially important to refuse to allow people who have an immune deficiency to change your baby's diapers.

Be aware that most doctors recommend not giving your child aspirin following the live polio vaccine, because aspirin use has been associated with Reye's syndrome when a child is ill with a virus. A "killed" polio vaccine is also available, but it is not thought to be as effective as the live vaccine.

The concept of "herd immunity" is based on the belief that if *most* people in a community are immune to a disease, an epidemic can be prevented. However, those in favor of 100 percent vaccination do not seem to recognize the fact that not *everyone* who receives a vaccine for a particular disease will be totally immune to this disease. The belief that allowing one person to be free from immunity will endanger everyone is without validity.

Medical care is an individual question in a free country. Medical practice has a tendency to follow traditions long after they are useful. Vaccinations should be a question for each individual to answer. Only then will we be free to be healthy.

VACCINATIONS AND INFORMED CHOICE
BY MAGDA KRANCE

Magda Krance is a public relations associate for Lyric Opera of Chicago. As a freelance journalist, her work has appeared in Time, People, *the* New York Times, *the* Chicago Tribune, American Health, Parenting, Spy, EcoTraveler, *and several other publications. She lives with her husband, Steve Leonard, and young son, Casimir, in Chicago, Illinois. "Vaccinations and Informed Choice" first appeared in* Mothering, *no. 39 (Summer 1991).*

My husband and I were uneasy as our son approached the age of two months, the time for his first diphtheria-pertussis-tetanus (DPT) shot. I had done extensive research on the subject of vaccinations the year before, and the tales of alleged adverse reactions to the pertussis component—brain damage, convulsions, physical handicaps, death—were horrifying, as were the suggestions that more subtle side effects, such as hyperactivity, learning disabilities, epilepsy, chronic allergies, asthma, vision and hearing problems, and even eczema might be linked to the inoculations. Additionally, the idea of someone injecting syringes full of toxoids and chemicals, including trace amounts of aluminum, formaldehyde (a mercury derivative), hydrochloric acid, and charcoal into our healthy son was disturbing.

Also distressing, though, was the newspaper article about the uninoculated children in a Buffalo, New York, family who came down with whooping cough, as pertussis is also known—a serious, sometimes fatal disease, especially for infants under six months of age. The violent coughing fits can cause babies to turn blue and to suffocate. *Uncomplicated* cases can last up to ten weeks, and hospitalization and intensive respiratory therapy are usually necessary. Although the children in the Buffalo family survived, the experience was no doubt as guilt-provoking for the parents, who had elected to forgo the shots, as it was physically traumatic for the kids, who had no say in the matter.

Of course, one seldom sees articles about the millions of children who have been vaccinated without incident, and the smaller number who have not had the shots but still remained healthy, or have become ill and recovered without complications. As frightening as the horror stories are about children who have been injured by vaccines, it is important to remember that they do not reflect the experience of the vast majority.

Generally, the risk of vaccine injury appears to be relatively low, although it is difficult to say exactly how low for several reasons: some possible pertussis reactions may be misdiagnosed as sudden infant death syndrome; the reporting of vaccine injuries and the correlation of them to vaccine batch numbers have not been comprehensive over the years; and the manifestations of the alleged effects may occur after children have been exposed to other agents that cause similar problems, making it difficult for parents or medical professionals to connect, and especially to prove, cause and effect.

Even though *any* possibility of vaccine injury can be alarming to parents, it is essential to keep the inoculation controversy in perspective. Children are at far greater risk of accidental death every day in the bathtub or the family car than they are from becoming ill as a result of inoculations. Because most of the US population has been vaccinated, and because sanitation conditions are so much better than in previous times, the hazard of exposure is also very low.

Although it is not quite a Sophie's choice, still the decisions about inoculations that face parents can be agonizing. Because of societal pressures, parents sometimes feel that they have no choice at all, since proof of vaccination is required before children are admitted to school, and this often applies to daycare centers as well. We want to take it on faith that vaccinations are safe; the idea, after all, is to protect our children, not to harm them. Besides, most of us got the full battery of obligatory inoculations when we were children, and most of us turned out fine. Moreover, although most of us born before the measles-mumps-rubella vaccine was developed got itchy or chipmunk-cheeked, we also received sympathy and attention and got to stay in bed and watch TV. For the most part those childhood illnesses seemed like a tolerable rite of passage, at least in the clean, comfortable circumstances of my home. In impoverished, unsanitary settings, though, they can be lethal.

In recent years, there have been several outbreaks of measles and whooping cough around the country. These incidents have been accompanied by urgent drives for universal vaccination, warnings of the dire consequences of exposure to the diseases, and reassurances that studies have conclusively shown the pertussis vaccine to be safe. At the same time, dozens of heartrending stories about children who have been allegedly injured by vaccines (as well as their heartbroken, financially ruined parents) have appeared on television and in consumer publications over the past decade, causing increasing numbers of parents, and even some medical professionals, to question the safety of the pertussis vaccine and the wisdom of mandatory vaccination programs (which have been canceled in most Western European countries).

Currently both proponents and opponents of the pertussis vaccine are armed with arsenals of persuasive rhetoric and manipulated statistics. It is difficult to know which side to trust when the issue is as emotionally charged as your child's health and future. Should you trust the physicians and public health officials who insist that there is no proven link between the pertussis vaccine and brain damage, that the benefits of vaccination in general far outweigh the risks, that epidemics would sweep the country and harm vastly more children if the inoculations were not mandatory, that society's interests outweigh those of the individual, and that the few children who may be injured or killed by vaccines should be considered unfortunate but necessary "altruists"? Or should you trust those who oppose compulsory vaccination, who counter that some inoculations can cause injury and death, that they do not necessarily confer immunity (many of the teenagers who contracted measles in the recent outbreaks had been vaccinated), and that they should be a matter of personal choice?

There are no easy answers. Informed choice and consent are essential to safeguard your child's health. Parents have to be smart health consumers. The best path to follow is to personally investigate the pros and cons of vaccination in the context of your child's own medical history. Know all the options and ramifications before you decide whether you want your child to have any, some, or all of the recommended vaccinations. Find out what each shot contains and what the risks are of both the disease and the inoculation. For detailed information on vaccine ingredients, side effects, and contraindications (conditions in which a vaccine should not be given), check the *Physicians' Desk Reference* in the reference section of the library or ask to see your pharmacist's copy. A useful source of information on infectious diseases is the American Academy of Pediatrics' (AAP) *Red Book*; ask to see your physician's copy during your next office visit.

Granted, it is not easy to be well-informed; it takes persistence and time. Pamphlets promoting vaccination are ubiquitously available at schools and clinics, but information from those opposing vaccinations is more difficult to find. Concerned parents have to seek it out in medical reference books, in several books on the subject, and in newsletters and pamphlets distributed by ad hoc groups and alternative health organizations. If you have time to read only one book, read Harris L. Coulter and Barbara Loe Fisher's *DPT: A Shot in the Dark* (New York: Harcourt Brace Jovanovich, 1985), a remarkable work that blends personal stories with solid scientific research and reporting. Remember, however, that all information provided by either side has to be taken with a grain of salt.

Before making decisions regarding vaccinations, it may also be helpful to speak to people who have firsthand experience with the vaccines. Although their opinions will vary, they may provide a broader context in which to make judgments. Robert Daum, MD, professor of pediatrics and head of pediatric infectious diseases at the University of Chicago, and member of the AAP's committee on infectious diseases, approves of:

> ... *consumer awareness and education regarding the effects and side effects of all medical interventions. It's wonderful to have parents who seek information about the interventions being offered to their children. You can get a parent working with you. But I am also strongly provaccine. I believe that preventive medicine saves great anguish and suffering from the diseases the vaccines are designed to prevent. Polio and smallpox are gone only because immunizations have gotten rid of them. Immunization is such an important preventive medicine strategy.*

He notes with alarm that because of increased reports of vaccine injuries,

> ... *the risk-benefit analysis as perceived by society has changed. With whooping cough, you have a disease that used to kill young babies, and you have a vaccine that for many years was perceived as safe. Then a television show does an exposé on DPT ["DPT Vaccine Roulette" was broadcast by NBC in 1982], and suddenly it's perceived as unsafe, the lawsuits go through the roof, and public acceptance of the*

vaccine goes down. I've seen the diseases, I've seen the burden, and I feel good about recommending immunizations.

As an example of the opposite viewpoint, Kathi Williams believes her learning-disabled son suffered an adverse reaction to his fourth DPT shot nine years ago—an event that coincided with the televising of "DPT Vaccine Roulette." She and others who called the station after seeing the program were put in touch with each other; they subsequently formed a support and watchdog group, Dissatisfied Parents Together (DPT), which lobbies for safer vaccination programs and which now operates the National Vaccine Information Center. "Our concern is that the AAP and CDC want to prevent disease at all costs, the 'costs' being some children," Williams says. "It's a war on disease, but the 'soldiers' are the children. When it's your child, the risks are 100 percent—there are no benefits."

Thanks in part to intense lobbying by DPT and other groups concerned about the safety of the pertussis vaccine, the National Childhood Vaccine Injury Act passed in 1986 and was enacted in 1988. It requires doctors to record the batch, lot number, and date of all vaccines given and to report adverse reactions to the CDC.

If you decide to have your child vaccinated, be sure to get a copy of the completed form for each injection from the doctor for your own records. You will need the information in the unlikely event that your child suffers an adverse reaction that should be reported, such as high fever (over 103°), acute diarrhea or vomiting, convulsions, seizures, extended high-pitched screaming, paralysis, unconsciousness, or death. In the past, there was no systematic recording or reporting of such reactions, making it virtually impossible for parents whose children had allegedly been injured or killed by vaccines to link the events in court.

Most pediatricians now give parents a checklist of possible side effects to watch for following the DPT inoculation, the vaccine with the highest rate of adverse reactions because of the pertussis component. If such a list is not offered, ask for it. According to the CDC, convulsions (with or without fever) and shock occur in one in 1,750 doses of vaccine given, and permanent neurological damage—retardation, paralysis, spasticity—occurs in one out of 310,000 doses. It is recommended that each child receive five doses of the vaccine before entering school, and up to 20 million doses of DPT vaccine are given in the US each year.

"Recording data by 'immunization' is thoroughly illogical [because] incidence expressed in terms of shots does not correlate with incidence in terms of children," contend Harris L. Coulter and Barbara Loe Fisher in their book *DPT: A Shot in the Dark* (recently updated, reprinted, and available in paperback). "It is misleading to give results in terms of shots administered," Coulter and Fisher say. "It is not shots that run high fevers, develop convulsions, become mentally retarded, or die. This happens to children." The authors cite a 1978–1979 study of adverse reactions to the pertussis vaccine conducted by the University of California–Los Angeles and the Food and Drug Administration, reporting that of the 3.3 million children vaccinated every year in the US, within 48 hours nearly 8,500 have convulsions, nearly 8,500 undergo collapse, and about 16,000 have episodes of high-pitched (encephalitic) screaming, which may indicate central nervous system irritation.

Some other good points to consider are made by J. Anthony Morris, PhD, a former government virologist who was fired in 1976 because he was critical of the swine flu vaccination program, which produced a large number of injuries and lawsuits, many still unsettled to this day. Morris remarks, "I'm all for inoculation programs for measles, mumps, and rubella, but I'm against placing faulty vaccines on the market. The early measles vaccines were clearly faulty; the current pertussis vaccine is clearly faulty and could be improved." (A safer pertussis vaccine has been in use for several years in Japan and became available in the US in the 1990s.)

Another problem, Morris says, is the premise and practice of mass inoculation:

When a vaccine is mandated, then not only do the manufacturers get careless, but the pediatrician administering the vaccine gets careless. When you have mass vaccination programs . . . carelessness comes into play, and you give a vaccine to a child who shouldn't receive it at that time because of illness. . . . Carelessness is almost inescapable in mass vaccination programs, where you're concerned with the benefit that society derives, not with what happens to the individual child. It's like the army, but it's children being hurt, not soldiers. I'm against mass inoculations. Each child should be considered as an individual. If that were the case, you would reduce to an insignificant [level] the number of cases of brain damage and death from the DPT vaccine.

If you decide you do not want your child to receive some of the inoculations, ask your physician to write a medical exemption. Some will; others may refuse to treat your child at all unless you agree to all the shots. Find out what vaccinations your state requires; the requirements and exemptions vary from state to state. Some states accept a philosophical or "personal belief" exemption as well as a religious exemption. Religious exemptions are accepted in most states and are not necessarily restricted to members of "recognized" religions, such as Christian Scientists, Jehovah's Witnesses, and Seventh-day Adventists, who typically do invoke the exemption. Check carefully with your own state health department for the latest legislative changes.

In addition to obtaining sufficient information, communication is important in determining the correct course of action regarding vaccination; to protect your child's health, two-way communication with your doctor is not a luxury but a necessity. Ask lots of questions rather than blindly submitting to a pediatrician's authority as so many people are conditioned to do. Do not let your doctor tell you that he or she knows what is best for your child without giving reasons for such decisions. Good doctors should have no problem with requests for explanations, but less competent ones may get defensive or angry. If that happens, find another doctor.

Physicians, too, have to ask questions to be sure that each child's health and family medical history do not pose the risk of a serious adverse reaction. You want your pediatrician to ask, and you need to be able to answer, the following questions: Has the child been sick lately? Is there currently any infection or fever? Is there a history of convulsions or neurological illness in the family? A history of allergies in the family? A history of drug use that might cause neurological problems in the child, such as maternal cocaine use during pregnancy? Was the child premature or did the child have a low birth weight? Are there any immune system problems? Has the child shown an allergic reaction to milk? Was there any cerebral irritation or injury at birth? Has the child had a bad reaction to a previous inoculation?

Unfortunately, such communication with doctors is sometimes

difficult because families may be forced by HMOs to abruptly change caregivers, others are dependent on overcrowded public clinics, and physicians are pressured by too many patients and too little time. Consequently, it can be hard to make sure your pediatrician knows that your baby is just getting over a cold, or that epilepsy runs in the family, or whatever the mitigating factors may be.

I was braced for a disagreement with our baby's doctor when we took him in for his two-month exam. Before I could open my mouth, though, she announced, "I don't want to give him the pertussis component, because of the seizure he had after he was born." Indeed, he had had focal seizures in one hand when he was less than a day old and had spent the next few days in intensive care until it was determined that my long labor had caused a tiny hemmorhage to form under his skull. Our pediatrician had made the correct decision regarding the pertussis vaccine, considering our baby's short but dramatic medical history. We were greatly relieved, and our child suffered no ill effects from the diphtheria-tetanus shot he received.

At present our knowledge about the effectiveness and dangers of vaccines is also being revised according to new data, some of which can be confusing. Although the medical community uses the words *inoculation, vaccination,* and *immunization* interchangeably, with *immunization* the favored term, vaccinations given to older children and young adults have not necessarily guaranteed immunity. In Houston, where 1,743 cases of measles were confirmed between October 1988 and June 1989, more than 50 percent of the cases were considered unpreventable, even though most in that group had been previously "immunized."

It is also advisable to be current regarding the latest information about the effectiveness of various vaccines, since that information is updated and revised according to new medical research and the experiences of those who have been vaccinated. For example, the measles vaccine administered during the 1970s lacked a stabilizer and consequently lost its efficacy if left unrefrigerated; a stabilizer was not added until 1980. Another example is the fact that until the mid-1970s babies were vaccinated against measles between the ages of nine and 12 months. However, subsequently it was discovered that maternal antibodies in the baby interfered with the vaccine's effectiveness, which is why the measles shot is now administered to children when they are 15 months old.

My pediatrician's office recently faxed me several pages of information from the AAP's *Red Book* about pertussis symptoms and treatment. Included was the estimate that vaccine efficacy for young children who have received at least three doses of DPT vaccine is 80 percent. The report also said that vaccine-induced "immunity" lasts for about three years and then gradually diminishes. Does that mean that 20 percent of vaccinated children may come down with whooping cough if they are exposed? Does it mean that all vaccinated individuals have a 20 percent chance of getting whooping cough? And if so, does it still make sense to vaccinate?

Anthony Morris, too, thinks parents should have the final say. "It's not necessary to mandate a program whose benefits are overwhelming," he says. "Logistically, it's easier to carry out mandatory inoculations, but democracy is not supposed to be easy. If you give a parent all the facts about the benefits and risks of vaccination, then the parent will make a wise choice. The parent will almost invariably say yes to vaccination voluntarily."

IMMUNIZATIONS AND INFORMED CONSENT
BY CAROL MILLER

Carol Miller is a public health consultant who has been living in northern New Mexico for over 20 years. She received a master's in public health in health education from the University of California at Berkeley and has postgraduate education in bioethics at Georgetown University. In 1993, Miller served as a presidential appointee to the White House Health Care Task Force headed by Hillary Rodham Clinton. She was New Mexico's Green Party nominee for congress in the 1997 election to replace Bill Richardson, Ambassador to the UN. An earlier version of "Immunizations and Informed Consent" appeared in Mothering, *no. 26 (Winter 1983).*

This article is not a scientific analysis of the information available about immunizations. It describes the research I have done and also teaches how to do computer searches for information, but primarily it shares the conclusions I have drawn about current US immunization policy after five years of studying the question.

I first began to research the issue of immunization in 1976 because of the swine flu vaccine. I was in Berkeley at the School of Public Health studying for a master's degree, and all of our classes emphasized the importance of the swine flu vaccine. When it became apparent that the vaccine was not only a total failure but was also a health hazard and killer, there was a great deal of embarrassment among the vaccine proponents on the faculty.

My interest in immunizations has continued since then, and I have researched the issue in numerous medical journals. I feel compelled to write this article to help parents sift through the vast number of conflicting reports in order to decide whether or not they should immunize their children.

LAWS ABOUT HEALTH

The worst thing about the US immunization policy is that it is law. In 49 states it is mandatory for children to be immunized in order to attend school. Wyoming is the only state without such a law, but that is because it has the highest *voluntary* immunization rate in the country. There are schedules of specific immunizations by certain ages that *must* be met by all children . . . or must they?

It is possible for parents to file as conscientious objectors with their state health department, although this choice is not advertised. Several people I know who are conscientious objectors state that it is their "God-given right to refuse to immunize their child." Any lesser statement is unacceptable legally. For example, it is unacceptable legally to say, "I read 25 articles in medical journals, three newspaper articles, and saw on the *Today* show that the pertussis vaccine has serious side effects, and for this reason I don't want my child to have the pertussis vaccine." Such a statement is not reason enough from a legal standpoint to refuse to immunize your child against pertussis. This can be a serious problem with immunization policy; in order to legally refuse any single immunization it may be necessary to be opposed to all immunizations on religious grounds. (See State Exemptions, p. 306). Scientific evidence against the effectiveness of particular immunizations is insufficient. A court case may be necessary to test this discrepancy.

THE SCIENTIFIC EVIDENCE

The particular computer search I did turned up 161 articles about health problems associated with immunizations, and all of these articles were only for the years 1980 and 1981. There is a tremendous debate in the medical world about the dangers of immunizations, but none of this information is leaked to the public until a large number of tragedies occur. The scientific evidence exists against some immunizations, but the political and economic reasons for their continuation remain stronger than these facts.

INFORMED CONSENT

Informed consent is an elusive concept, one which is often resolved only in courts of law. In the area of immunizations there is almost no such thing as informed consent. Parents must sign a release of liability to the drug company when giving their child the polio vaccine, because so many victims have suffered from the treatment that the company is forced to protect itself. There is very little accurate information being presented about the other vaccines.

What is known about vaccines is an entirely different story from what is told. Healthcare consumers should insist on reading the package inserts that come with vaccines. Many medical professionals have never read these inserts and therefore are not able to tell you that there are some conditions that make vaccines health hazards.

Although the actual package inserts detail the very serious complications of immunizations, the federal Centers for Disease Control (the agency in charge of national immunization policy) sent a letter to all of the state immunization officers that read:

Vaccine Side Effects—Vaccines are among our safest and most reliable medicines. However, vaccines, like many medicines, can cause side effects. These are usually mild and brief, such as low fever, sore arm, slight rash, or irritability after taking the shot. Very rarely, they are serious. For this reason, vaccines should be given only by physicians or other qualified persons and only to those who need them.

I would like to contrast this official policy statement of the federal government with a letter I received from a mother as a result of an article I wrote for *New Age* magazine entitled "The Truth about Immunizations" (September 1980). I received more letters in response to this article than I have to anything else I have ever written. I am overwhelmed by the concern of people about this issue:

Dear Carol,
Outrage seems like an oversimplified word to use in expressing our feeling when our perfectly healthy (then 15½-month-old) son received a measles-mumps-rubella shot. Not only did the health department flyer explaining the vaccine and its reactions clearly misinform us, but the nurse who administered the vaccine was just as ignorant. After less than 24 hours our warm, smiling, energetic kid turned into a zombie, burning a fever of close to 105°! The drug company says a reaction to the shot may occur from ten to 12 days within the initial administering period. Well, somebody ought to set those folks straight and tell them how our child suffered for close to four days from the vaccine and, on top of that, on the fifth day broke out in a measly rash that lasted one and a half weeks.

Mothering published a similar letter from a mother whose emotion haunted me as she stated, "When I signed the consent paper saying I knew that one in a million has a postvaccinal encephalitis reaction, I did not possibly believe that my son would be that *one!*"

This letter was also about a reaction to the MMR vaccine.

I could quote many other letters like this and also many more positive ones from parents all over the country who have refused to immunize their children. These are satisfied parents with healthy children who feel that proper diet, breastfeeding, and other lifestyle choices have helped to make their children healthier than immunizations could.

Mothering has printed many articles and letters in back issues about the immunization question, but the majority of parents in this country have never learned about the possible hazards. It seems that an organization should be started to educate parents about vaccines and to lobby for their legal right to informed consent.

WHAT IS AN IMMUNIZATION MADE OF?

Most parents who are trying to feed their children properly would not let them eat a food that contains any of the many ingredients of immunizations. Some of the ingredients in vaccines are phenol (carbolic acid), formaldehyde (a known cancer-causing agent that is commonly used to embalm corpses), mercury (a toxic heavy metal), alum (a preservative), aluminum phosphate (a toxic substance used in deodorants), acetone (a solvent used in fingernail polish remover, very volatile, crosses placenta easily), glycerin, sodium chloride, pig or horse blood, cow pox pus, rabbit brain tissues, dog kidney tissue, monkey kidney tissue, chicken or duck egg protein, and other decomposing protein.

The scientific theory behind immunizations is that by receiving a small dose of a virus or bacteria, the body will develop enough immunities to the small dose to protect it from coming down with that specific disease on a larger scale. The animal parts ingredients in immunizations are used to grow the viruses that are later injected into children. The other toxic ingredients are added in either the chemical production of the vaccine or as preservatives.

FOREIGN TRAVEL AND VACCINATION

Many people wonder about immunizing their children before traveling to a foreign country. This is a confusing issue with many complicating factors. The most complicating is that when traveling it is much more difficult for parents to maintain control over their children's environment than it is at home. Food and water may be contaminated, and all living conditions may be unhealthier than at home.

In spite of these difficulties, many people travel without receiving immunizations. One of the largest groups to do so is Christian Scientists. Thousands of Christian Scientists travel outside the US every year, and their religion forbids them to immunize. The Amish and Mennonites are examples of other religious sects that do not believe in vaccination.

HOW TO MAKE VACCINATION DECISIONS

I stated earlier that this article was not going to be a scientific analysis of immunization. Nor is it a guide to which immunizations to give. This is because of my basic premise that parents have to make decisions for themselves about whether or not to immunize their children, and against which diseases. However, I can offer ideas for parents about how to research this issue and where to go for more information. Such information will range from totally provaccination to totally opposed. I am presenting a middle path that encourages parents to learn what they can, ask lots of questions, and then decide what to do for their own children.

Demand informed consent not only in the matter of immunization, but in any health matter that confronts you. This means you should not agree to any health procedure until all of your questions have been answered to your satisfaction. This is not an easy job, and very few health professionals will help you in your search for answers, but it is a crucial process.

After a while you will be wondering how to know who to believe. Trust your instincts. Don't let guilt prod you into a decision you are uncomfortable with. Locate people whose advice you respect, whether it is newspaper-column physician Robert Mendelsohn or "Dear Abby." Magazines such as *Mothering, New Age, East West Journal,* and *Yoga Journal* all try to present minority opinions about health issues.

HOW TO USE A COMPUTER TO SEARCH FOR INFORMATION

People are drowning in statistics. It seems these days that *any* issue elicits pro and con statistics, and many of us find that too much information can often confuse decision making rather than facilitate it.

Computers have contributed to this because of their incredible information and retrieval capabilities. More people need to learn how to get information from a computer in order to sort out the amount of information with which we are barraged. When I am confused with conflicting information about a health issue, I conduct a computer search to help make a decision. It is very easy and not too expensive.

There are two ways to do a computer search. With the right tools a search can easily be done on a home or office computer, or the search can be done at a facility with computer search capabilities.

Do-It-Yourself Computer Research

Due to improvements in computer technology and the large number of people who now use computers on a regular basis, obtaining health information is easier than ever. Anyone with a home computer, a modem, and the right software can directly access a variety of electronic databases and do his or her own search. People who have a continuing interest in healthcare issues may want to learn how to do their own searches.

The best software to use for medical data searching is GRATEFUL MED, developed and distributed by the National Library of Medicine at the National Institutes of Health. This software is very easy to use, quite inexpensive, and is available in Macintosh and PC versions. Information about GRATEFUL MED can be obtained from the National Library of Medicine, public information, 800-272-4787; and from Medlars Services, 800-638-8480.

Computer Research at a Facility

The second option in computer research is to have it done at a facility. The steps involved in doing such a search follow.

Locate a Facility

Computers that link into health information are located in medical school libraries, hospital libraries, large city libraries, other schools, and at various governmental agencies.

The On-line Search

Even though it is possible to set up a search over the telephone and receive the results in the mail, if at all possible it is best to be present for the on-line search. "On-line" means that you are directly linked to the computer and can ask questions, change topics, and see answers immediately as they print out. For example, I did an on-line MEDLINE search on immunization using as key words *failure, poisoning,* and *toxicity*. The computer printed out that there were 1,061 citations. This was too many for the scope of this article, so I narrowed it to *poisoning* and *toxicity* and found that there were 161 citations.

I could have 40 of them printed on-line, so the computer then printed the titles, journals, and issues of the journals on a list for me. This concluded the on-line search. There are a number of other data banks available besides MEDLINE; for example, CANLIT for cancer research and TOXLINE for toxicology.

THE OFF-LINE SEARCH

Off-line searches are done on specific retrieval requests and are much cheaper. My on-line search printout with 40 citations cost $9.00, but to have the remaining 121 titles printed out off-line cost only $1.80. Off-line searches are not immediate and may take up to a week.

THE ACTUAL RESEARCH

Using the same example, the research for this article, I divided the information from the MEDLINE search into categories by type of vaccine. Twenty-two percent of the articles discussed poisoning and toxicity associated with the pertussis immunization, 13 percent with rubella immunization, 9 percent with polio, 7 percent with smallpox, and 6 percent with measles. I decided that 29 of the 121 articles sounded very interesting, so before I looked them up in the journals, I did a second off-line search with the identification numbers of those 29 articles in order to have the abstracts (introductions) printed out to study.

This process saves hundreds of research hours. As a health professional I have learned that this journal information is the only data considered "worthy" of debate by doctors, so for me it is impossible to skip this step. As a healthcare consumer I have found that the computer search can help me to get better care and change physicians' minds so that others can get better care as well.

CONSTITUTIONAL RIGHTS AND IMMUNIZATION
BY CAROL MILLER

Officially, immunization policy in the US comes from two primary sources: the American Academy of Pediatrics and the federal Centers for Disease Control. These two groups issue guidelines and policies that are used by most healthcare providers and state health departments. However, in reality most immunization policy is either developed by or developed in connection with the vaccine manufacturers. There are varied approaches to the implementation of these policies among states and other public health agencies. Some states and public school districts are much more accepting of parents who object to immunization than others.

Parents in many locales have protested that their rights and their children's rights have been infringed upon due to overzealous immunization policies. Children have been threatened with expulsion or ousted from schools for their beliefs—even when these children belonged to a religion that prohibits immunization. There have been cases where social service agencies have taken children away from their parents, called these parents unfit, and forced the children to be immunized. It is sad to report that in many places, authorities treat people who disagree with mainstream immunization policies as if they have no constitutional rights to choose which medical services they want. Those policies are challenged in courts, and various jurisdictions adjudicate them differently.

What interest group has the most rights when it comes to immunizations? It is not surprising that the drug manufacturers have reserved most of these rights for themselves. They develop and manufacture a product that has a gigantic automatic market. And they are completely protected from liability by US taxpayers.

The case of the pertussis vaccine provides a good illustration of this situation. In the past, numerous children have had adverse reactions to the pertussis vaccine—so many that articles about such cases appeared frequently in newspapers, and parents of affected children were guests on TV talk shows. As a result, many parents began to fear the pertussis vaccine. Then the manufacturer slowed production to a standstill, and suddenly there was a shortage. Rather than reassess the national pertussis immunization policy, the federal government agreed to absolve manufacturers of any liability and established a Vaccine Injury Trust Fund administered by the Department of Health and Human Services (DHHS). This fund provides tax dollars to compensate people injured by vaccines. However, even though the taxpayers now pay for vaccine-caused death and injury, there has been no reduction in the price charged for vaccines. In the 1992 DHHS budget, the vaccine injury program received $82.5 million. This amount is over and above the millions in the Vaccine Injury Trust Fund. The question remains, if the government has to pay so many millions of dollars every year to compensate people injured by vaccines, why can't parents have the right to *not* immunize their children?

PHILOSOPHICAL QUESTIONS

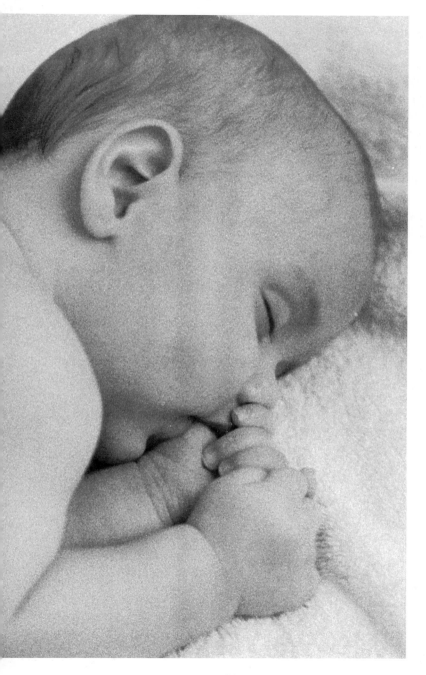

Immunizations: The Other Side

By Richard Moskowitz

Richard Moskowitz, MD, received his undergraduate degree from Harvard University and his medical degree from New York University before studying homeopathy with George Vithoulkas in Athens, Greece. He served as president of the National Center for Homeopathy in Washington, DC, from 1985 to 1986, and is the author of Homeopathic Medicines for Pregnancy and Childbirth, *published in 1992 by North Atlantic Press. A contributing editor to* Mothering, *Moskowitz currently practices classical homeopathy in Watertown, Massachusetts.* "Immunizations: The Other Side" *is an abridged version of an article that originally appeared in the* Journal of the American Institute of Homeopathy *(1983). An earlier version of this article was published in* Mothering, *no. 31 (Spring 1984).*

See also "Unvaccinated Children," 158, and "Vaccination: A Sacrament of Modern Medicine," 168, by Moskowitz.

The growing refusal of parents to vaccinate their children is seldom articulated or taken seriously. The fact is that we have been taught to accept vaccination as a sort of involuntary communion, a sacrament of our own participation in the unrestricted growth of scientific and industrial technology, utterly heedless of the long-term consequences to the health of our own species, not to mention the balance of nature as a whole. For that reason alone, the other side of the case urgently needs to be heard.

Are Vaccines Effective?

There is widespread agreement that, in the time period since the common vaccines were introduced, we have seen a remarkable decline in the incidence and severity of the corresponding natural infections. But the customary assumption that the decline is *attributable* to the vaccines remains unproven and continues to be seriously questioned by eminent authorities in the field. The incidence and severity of whooping cough had already begun to decline precipitously long before the pertussis vaccine was introduced,[1] a fact that led the epidemiologist C. C. Dauer to remark, as far back as 1943:

If mortality [from pertussis] continues to decline at the same rate during the next 15 years, it will be extremely difficult to show statistically that [pertussis immunization] had any effect in reducing mortality from whooping cough.[2]

Much the same is true not only of diphtheria and tetanus, but also of tuberculosis, cholera, typhoid, and other common scourges of a bygone era, which began to disappear toward the end of the 19th century, perhaps partly in response to improvements in public health and sanitation, but in any case long before antibiotics, vaccines, or any specific medical measures designed to eradicate them.[3]

Reflections such as these led the great microbiologist René Dubos to observe that microbial diseases have their own natural history, independent of drugs and vaccines, in which asymptomatic infection and symbiosis are far more common than overt disease:

It is barely recognized, but nevertheless true, that animals and plants, as well as men, can live peacefully with their most notorious microbial enemies. The world is obsessed by the fact that poliomyelitis can kill and maim several thousand unfortunate victims every year. But more extraordinary is the fact that millions upon millions of young people become infected by polio viruses, yet suffer no harm from the infection. The dramatic episodes of conflict between men and microbes are what strike the mind. What is less readily apprehended is the more common fact that infection can occur without producing disease.[4]

The principal evidence that the vaccines are effective actually dates from the more recent period, during which time the dreaded polio epidemics of the 1940s and 1950s have never reappeared in developed countries, and measles, mumps, and rubella, which even a generation ago were among the most common diseases of childhood, have become far less prevalent, at least in their classic acute forms, since the triple MMR vaccine was introduced into common use.

Yet how the vaccines actually accomplish these changes is not nearly as well understood as most people like to think. The disturbing possibility that they act in some other way than by producing a genuine immunity is suggested by the fact that the diseases in ques-

tion have continued to break out even in highly immunized populations, and that in such cases the observed differences in incidence
and severity between immunized and unimmunized persons have
tended to be far less dramatic than expected, and in some cases not
measurably significant at all.

In a recent British outbreak of whooping cough, for example,
even fully immunized children contracted the disease in fairly large
numbers, and the rates of serious complications and death were
reduced only slightly.[5] In another recent outbreak of pertussis, 46 of
the 85 fully immunized children studied eventually contracted the
disease.[6]

In 1977, 34 new cases of measles were reported on the campus
of UCLA, in a population that was supposedly 91 percent immune,
according to careful serological testing.[7] Another 20 cases of measles
were reported in the Pecos, New Mexico, area within a period of a few
months in 1981, and at least 75 percent of the people involved had
been fully immunized, some quite recently.[8] A survey of sixth graders
in a well-immunized urban community revealed that about 15 percent of this group are still susceptible to rubella, a figure essentially
identical with that of the prevaccine era.[9]

Finally, although the overall incidence of typical acute measles
in the US has dropped sharply from about 400,000 cases annually in
the early 1960s to about 30,000 cases by 1974 to 1976, the death rate
has remained exactly the same;[10] and, with the peak incidence now
occurring in adolescents and young adults, the risk of pneumonia
and demonstrable liver abnormalities has actually increased sub-
stantially, according to one recent study, to well over 3 percent and 20
percent, respectively.[11]

The simplest way to explain these discrepancies would be to
postulate that the vaccines confer only partial or temporary immunity, which sounds reasonable enough, given the fact that they are
either live viruses rendered less virulent by serial passage in tissue
culture, or bacteria or bacterial proteins that have been killed or
denatured by heat, such that they can still elicit an antibody
response but no longer initiate the full-blown disease.

Because the vaccine is a "trick," in the sense that it *stimulates*
the true or natural immune response developed in the course of
recovering from the actual disease, it is certainly realistic to expect
that such artificial immunity will in fact "wear off" quite easily, and

even require additional booster doses at regular intervals throughout life to maintain peak effectiveness.

Such an explanation would be disturbing enough for most people. Indeed, the basic fallacy inherent in it is painfully evident in the fact that there is no way to know how long this partial or temporary immunity will last in any given individual, or how often it will need to be restimulated, because the answers to these questions clearly depend on precisely the same individual variables that would have determined whether or how severely the same person, unvaccinated, would have contracted the disease in the first place.

In any case, a number of other observations suggest equally strongly that this simple explanation cannot be the correct one. First, a number of investigators have shown that when a person vaccinated against measles, for example, again becomes susceptible to it, even repeated booster doses will have little or no effect.[12]

Second, the vaccines do not act merely by producing pale or mild copies of the original disease; all of them also commonly produce a variety of symptoms of their own. Moreover, in some cases, these illnesses may be considerably more serious than the original disease, involving deeper structures, more vital organs, and less of a tendency to resolve spontaneously. Even more worrisome is the fact that they are almost always more difficult to recognize.

Thus in a recent outbreak of mumps in supposedly immune schoolchildren, several developed atypical symptoms, such as anorexia, vomiting, and erythematous rashes, without any parotid involvement (swollen glands), and the diagnosis required extensive serological testing to rule out other concurrent diseases.[13] The syndrome of "atypical measles" can be equally difficult to diagnose, even when it is thought of,[14] which suggests that it is often overlooked entirely. In some cases, atypical measles can be much more severe than the regular kind, with pneumonia, petechiae, edema, and severe pain,[15] and likewise often goes unsuspected.

In any case, it seems virtually certain that other vaccine-related syndromes will be described and identified if only we take the trouble to look for them, and that the ones we are aware of so far represent only a very small part of the problem. But even these few make it less and less plausible to assume that the vaccines produce a normal, healthy immunity that lasts for some time but then wears off, leaving the patient miraculously unharmed and unaffected by the experience.

THE INDIVIDUAL VACCINES RECONSIDERED

Next I wish to consider each of the vaccines on an individual basis in relation to the infectious diseases from which they are derived.

The MMR is composed of attenuated live measles, mumps, and rubella viruses administered in a single intramuscular injection at about 15 months of age. Subsequent reimmunization is no longer recommended except for young women of childbearing age, in whom the risk of congenital rubella syndrome (CRS) is thought to warrant it, even though the effectiveness of reimmunization is questionable at best.

Prior to the vaccine era, measles, mumps, and rubella were reckoned among the routine childhood diseases, which most schoolchildren contracted before the age of puberty, and from which nearly all recovered with permanent, lifelong immunity and with no complications or sequelae.

However, such diseases were not always so harmless. Measles in particular can be a devastating disease when a population encounters it *for the first time*. Its importation from Spain, for instance, undoubtedly contributed to Cortés's conquest of the great Aztec empire; whole villages were depopulated by epidemics of measles and smallpox, leaving only a small remnant of cowed, superstitious warriors to face the bearded conquistadors from across the sea.[16] In more recent outbreaks among isolated, primitive peoples, the case fatality rate from measles averaged 20 to 30 percent.[17]

In these so-called virgin-soil epidemics, not only measles but polio and many other similar diseases take their highest toll of death and serious complications among adolescents and young adults— healthy and vigorous people in the prime of life—and leave relatively unharmed the group of children younger than puberty.[18]

This means that the evolution of a disease such as measles from a dreaded killer to an ordinary disease of childhood presupposes the development of nonspecific or "herd" immunity in young children, such that, when they are finally exposed to the disease, it activates defense mechanisms already prepared to receive it, resulting in the long incubation period and the usually benign, self-limited course.

Under these circumstances, the rationale for wanting to vaccinate young children against measles is limited to the fact that a very small number of deaths and serious complications have continued to occur, chiefly pneumonia, encephalitis, and the rare but dreaded subacute sclerosing panencephalitis (SSPE), a slow-virus disease with a reported incidence of one per 100,000 cases.[19] Pneumonia, by far the most common complication, is usually benign and self-limited, even without treatment;[20] and even in those rare cases in which bacterial pneumonia supervenes, adequate treatment is currently available.

By all accounts, then, the death rate from wild-type measles is very low, the incidence of serious sequelae is insignificant, and the general benefit to the child who recovers from the disease, and to his contacts and descendants, is very great. Consequently, even if the measles vaccine could be shown to reduce the risk of death or serious complications from the disease, it still could not justify the high probability of autoimmune diseases, cancer, and whatever else may result from the propagation of latent measles virus in human tissue culture for life.

The case for immunizing against mumps and rubella seems *a fortiori* even more tenuous, for exactly the same reasons. Mumps is also essentially a benign, self-limited disease in children before the age of puberty, and recovery from a single attack confers lifelong immunity. The principal complication is meningoencephalitis, mild or subclinical forms of which are relatively common, although the death rate is extremely low[21] and sequelae are rare.

The mumps vaccine is prepared and administered in much the same way as the measles vaccine, usually in the same injection, and the dangers associated with it are likewise comparable. Like measles, mumps is fast becoming a disease of adolescents and young adults,[22] age groups that tolerate the disease much less well. The chief complication is acute epididymo-orchitis, which occurs in 30 to 40 percent of the males affected past the age of puberty and usually results in atrophy of the testicle on the affected side;[23] but it also shows a strong tendency to attack the ovary and the pancreas.

For all of these reasons, the greatest favor we could do for our children would be to expose them all to the measles and mumps when they are young, which would not only protect them against contracting more serious forms of these diseases when they grow older, but would also greatly assist in their immunological maturation with minimal risk. I need hardly add that this is very close to the actual evolution of these diseases before the MMR vaccine was introduced.

The same discrepancy is evident in the case of rubella, or German measles, which in young children is a disease so mild that it frequently escapes detection,[24] but in older children and adults not infrequently produces arthritis, purpura, and other severe, systemic signs.[25] The main impetus for the development of the vaccine was certainly the recognition of the CRS resulting from damage to the developing embryo in utero during the first trimester of pregnancy,[26] and the relatively high incidence of CRS traceable to the rubella outbreak of 1964.

But here again we have an almost entirely benign, self-limited disease transformed by the vaccine into a considerably less benign disease of adolescents and young adults of reproductive age, which is ironically the group that most needs to be protected against it. Moreover, as with measles and mumps, the simplest and most effective way to prevent CRS would be to expose everybody to rubella in elementary school; reinfection does sometimes occur after recovery from rubella, but much less commonly than after vaccination.[27]

The equation looks somewhat different for the diphtheria and tetanus vaccines. First of all, both diphtheria and tetanus are serious, sometimes fatal diseases, even with the best of treatment; this is especially true of tetanus, which still carries a mortality rate of close to 50 percent.

Furthermore, these vaccines are not made from living diphtheria and tetanus organisms, but only from certain toxins elaborated by them. These poisonous substances are still highly antigenic, even after being inactivated by heat. Diphtheria and tetanus toxoids, therefore, do not protect against infections per se, but only against the systemic action of the original poisons, in the absence of which both infections are of minor importance clinically.

Consequently, it is easy to understand why parents might want their children protected against diphtheria and tetanus if safe and effective protection were available. Moreover, both vaccines have been in use for a long time, and the reported incidence of serious problems has remained very low, so there has never been much public outcry against them.

On the other hand, both diseases are quite readily controlled by simple sanitary measures and careful attention to wound hygiene; and, in any case, both have been steadily disappearing from the developing countries since long before the vaccines were introduced.

Diphtheria now occurs sporadically in the US, often in areas with significant reservoirs of unvaccinated children. But the claim that the vaccine is "protective" is once again belied by the fact that, when the disease does break out, the supposedly "susceptible" children are in fact no more likely to develop clinical diphtheria than their fully immunized contacts. In a 1969 outbreak in Chicago, for example, the Board of Health reported that 25 percent of the cases had been fully immunized and that another 12 percent had received one or more doses of the vaccine and showed serological evidence of full immunity; another 18 percent had been partly immunized, according to the same criteria.[28]

So once again we are faced with the probability that what the diphtheria toxoid has produced is not a genuine immunity to diphtheria at all, but rather some sort of chronic immune *tolerance* to it by harboring highly antigenic residues somewhere within the cells of the immune system, presumably with long-term suppressive effects on the immune mechanism generally.

This suspicion is further substantiated by the fact that all of the diphtheria-pertussis-tetanus (DPT) vaccines are alum-precipitated and preserved with thimerosal, an organomercury derivative, to prevent them from being metabolized too rapidly, so that the antigenic challenge will continue for as long as possible. The fact is that we do not know and have never even attempted to discover what actually becomes of these foreign substances once they are inside the human body.

Exactly the same problems complicate the record of the tetanus vaccine, which almost certainly has had at least some impact in reducing the incidence of tetanus in its classic acute form, yet presumably also survives for years or even decades as a potent foreign antigen within the body, with long-term incalculable effects on the immune system and elsewhere.

Whooping cough, much like diphtheria and tetanus, began to decline as a serious epidemiological threat long before the vaccine was introduced. Moreover, the vaccine has not been particularly effective, even according to its proponents, and the incidence of known side effects is disturbingly high.

The power of the pertussis vaccine to damage the central nervous system, for example, has received growing attention since Stewart and his colleagues reported an alarmingly high incidence of encephalopathy and severe convulsive disorders in British children, traceable to the vaccine.[29] My own cases suggest that hematological disturbances may be even more prevalent and that, in any case, the known complications almost certainly represent a small fraction of the total.

Pertussis is also extremely variable clinically, ranging in severity from asymptomatic, mild, or inapparent infections, which are quite common actually, to very rare cases in young infants less than five months of age, in whom the mortality rate is said to reach 40 percent.[30] Indeed, the disease is rarely fatal or even that serious in children over one year of age, and antibiotics have very little to do with the outcome.[31]

A good deal of the pressure to immunize at the present time thus seems to be attributable to the higher death rate in very young infants, which has led to the terrifying practice of giving this most clearly dangerous of the vaccines to infants at two months of age, when their mothers' milk would normally protect them from all infections about as well as can ever be done,[32] and when the effect on the still-developing blood and nervous systems could be catastrophic.

Poliomyelitis and the polio vaccines present an entirely different situation. The standard Sabin vaccine is trivalent, consisting of attenuated, live polioviruses of each of the three strains associated with poliomyelitis; but it is administered orally, in much the same way as the infection is acquired in nature. The oral, or noninjectable, route, which leaves the recipient free to develop a natural immunity at the normal portal of entry, that is, the gastrointestinal tract, would therefore appear to represent a considerable safety factor.

On the other hand, the wild-type poliovirus produces no symptoms whatsoever in over 90 percent of the people who contract it, even under epidemic conditions;[33] and of those people who do come down with recognizable clinical disease, perhaps only 1 or 2 percent ever progress to the full-blown neurological picture of poliomyelitis, with its characteristic lesions in the anterior horn cells of the spinal cord or medulla oblongata.[34]

Poliomyelitis thus presupposes peculiar conditions of susceptibility in the host, even a specific *anatomical* susceptibility, since even under epidemic conditions, the virulence of the poliovirus is so low, and the number of cases resulting in death or permanent disability is always remarkably small.[35]

Given the fact that the poliovirus was ubiquitous before the vaccine was introduced and could be found routinely in samples of city sewage wherever it was looked for,[36] it is evident that effective, natural immunity to poliovirus was already as close to being universal as it can ever be, and *a fortiori* no artificial substitute could ever equal or even approximate that result. Indeed, because the virulence of the poliovirus was so low to begin with, it is difficult to see what further attenuation of it could possibly accomplish, other than to abate as well the full vigor of the natural immune response to it.

For the fact remains that even the attenuated virus is still alive, and the people who were anatomically susceptible to it before are still susceptible to it now. This means, of course, that at least *some* of these same people will develop paralytic polio from the vaccine,[37] and that the others may still be harboring the virus in latent form, perhaps within those same cells.

The only obvious advantage of giving the vaccine, then, would be to introduce people to the virus when they are still infants, at a time when the virulence is normally lowest anyway;[38] but even this benefit could be more than offset by the danger of weakening the immune response. In any case, the whole matter is clearly one of enormous complexity and illustrates only too well the hidden dangers and miscalculations that are inherent in the virtually irresistible attempt to beat nature at her own game, to eliminate a problem that cannot be eliminated—namely the susceptibility to disease itself, and the *possibility* of sickness.

NOTES

1. E. Mortimer, "Pertussis Immunization," *Hospital Practice* (October 1980): 103.

2. Ibid., 105.

3. René Dubos, *The Mirage of Health* (New York: Harper & Row, 1959), 73.

4. Ibid., 74–75.

5. G. Stewart, "Vaccination against Whooping Cough: Efficiency vs. Risks," *The Lancet* (1977): 234.

6. *Medical Tribune* (10 January 1979): 1.

7. J. Cherry, "The New Epidemiology of Measles and Rubella," *Hospital Practice* (July 1980): 52–54.

8. Unpublished data from the New Mexico Health Department (private communication).

9. M. Lawless et al., "Rubella Susceptibility in Sixth-Graders," *Pediatrics* 65 (June 1980): 1086–1089.

10. See Note 7, 49.

11. *Infectious Diseases* (January 1982): 21.

12. See Note 7, 52.

13. *Family Practice News* (15 July 1980): 1.

14. J. Ferrante, "Atypical Symptoms? It Could *Still* Be Measles," *Modern Medicine* (30 September 1980): 76.

15. See Note 7, 53.

16. W. McNeill, *Plagues and Peoples* (New York: Doubleday, 1976), 184.

17. M. Burnet and D. White, *The Natural History of Infectious Disease* (Cambridge, MA: Harvard University Press, 1972), 16.

18. Ibid., 90, 121.

19. A. Steigman, "Slow Virus Infections," in Victor Vaughan and R. J. McKay, *Nelson Textbook of Pediatrics,* 11th ed. (Philadelphia: W. B. Saunders, Co., 1979), 937.

20. C. Phillips, in Vaughan et al., *Nelson Textbook of Pediatrics,* 860.

21. C. Phillips, "Mumps," in Vaughan et al., *Nelson Textbook of Pediatrics,* 891.

22. G. Hayden et al., "Mumps and Mumps Vaccine in the U.S.," *Continuing Education* (September 1979): 97.

23. See Note 21, 892.

24. C. Phillips, "Rubella," in Vaughan et al., *Nelson Textbook of Pediatrics,* 863.

25. Ibid., 862.

26. L. Glasgow and J. Overall, "Congenital Rubella Syndrome," in Vaughan et al., *Nelson Textbook of Pediatrics,* 483.

27. See Note 24, 865.

28. Cited in R. Mendelsohn, "The Truth about Immunizations," *The People's Doctor* (April 1978): 1.

29. See Note 5, 234.

30. R. Feigin, "Pertussis," in Vaughan et al., *Nelson Textbook of Pediatrics,* 769.

31. Ibid.

32. L. Barness, "Breast Feeding," in Vaughan et al., *Nelson Textbook of Pediatrics,* 191.

33. See Note 17, 91ff.

34. B. Davis et al., *Microbiology*, 2nd ed. (New York: Harper & Row, 1973), 1290ff.

35. Ibid., 1280.

36. See Note 17, 93.

37. V. Fulginiti, "Problems of Poliovirus Immunization," *Hospital Practice* (August 1980): 61–62.

38. See Note 17, 95

Bringing Vaccines into Perspective

By Harold E. Buttram

and John Chriss Hoffman

Harold E. Buttram, MD, is a general practitioner in addition to specializing in allergy and environmental medicine. He lives in Quakertown, Pennsylvania. John Chriss Hoffman studied for his PhD in microbiology at Catholic University in Washington, DC, and has been involved in the vaccination debate since 1978. "Bringing Vaccines into Perspective" first appeared in Mothering, *no. 34 (Winter 1985).*

At present there are two schools of thought concerning state and federally enforced vaccine programs for children and infants. On the one hand, an overwhelming majority of the members of the US medical and public health communities approve current vaccination programs; they accept the occasional toxic vaccine reaction in children as the price that must be paid for the seeming control gained over infectious diseases.

On the other hand, a small but growing minority of physicians and laypersons express concern about these vaccine programs, believing that the harm done from them may be far more extensive than generally recognized. All too often, the arguments of this latter group have lacked credibility because of a deficiency of concrete scientific evidence. In our opinion, this is now changing.

Increase in Allergic (Atopic) Disorders

Many practicing physicians in the US and Europe have made the observation that allergic and/or immunologic disorders in children are rapidly increasing. A review in *Modern Medicine* (May 1983) of an international allergy meeting in London stated: "There is little doubt that the incidence of allergic disorders has increased in recent years."[1] One prominent pediatrician has speculated that "there may be a relationship between immunization as a stress and the onset of some of the devastating array of symptoms I am seeing all the time in younger and younger children."[2]

In a survey conducted by Eaton,[3] the incidence of allergic problems in a sample population of women in England increased from 25 percent in 1974 to 32 percent in 1979; in men, reported allergic problems increased from 20 percent in 1974 to 27 percent in 1979. This represents an increased incidence of allergies of over 1 percent per year for the population surveyed. Atherton reported an alarming increase in atopic eczema in Great Britain.[4] Of a group of 12,555 children born in a single week in 1970, 12 percent were reported by their parents to have had atopic eczema by the age of five years,[5] more than twice the proportion reported in a similar study 12 years previously.

From our point of view, there may be several major factors in modern society that can potentially cause an immunologic weakening of our children. Such causes may include chemical pollution of air, food, and water; commercial formula feeding, instead of breast-feeding; excessive use of drugs in children and in mothers during pregnancy and lactation; and commercial food processing and devitalization.[6] In addition, current mass vaccination programs must be highly suspected as contributing to the increased incidence of allergic disorders.

LYMPHOCYTE ABNORMALITY FOLLOWING TETANUS BOOSTER SHOTS

A significant report appeared in the correspondence section of *The New England Journal of Medicine* (19 January 1984) entitled "Abnormal T-Lymphocyte Subpopulations in Healthy Subjects after Tetanus Booster Immunization."[7] The letter reported studies conducted to determine the effects of booster vaccination with tetanus toxoid on the ratio of the helper-to-suppressor T-lymphocytes of healthy adults. Indirect immunofluorescence evaluation of T-lymphocytes from blood samples taken before and after booster vaccination revealed a temporary drop, for each subject, in the helper/suppressor ratio after vaccination. The largest drop detected occurred between days 3 and 14 postvaccination, with four of the 11 subjects demonstrating ratios of 1.0 or less (normal values are in the range of 1.0 to 2.0). *The report pointed out that similar drops in helper/suppressor ratios of T-lymphocytes are characteristic of acquired immune deficiency syndrome (AIDS).*

The question is: Does a similar AIDS-like state occur in young children and infants following their receipt of multiple-vaccine regimens during the crucial period of their lives when their immune system is beginning to mature? Any suppression of the helper T-lymphocytes during this time, even of a transient nature, would most certainly be undesirable. What is known is that an AIDS-like reduced

T-lymphocyte ratio has been described in *young children* and may be the underlying cause of transient hypogammaglobulinemia (reduced level of protective immunoglobulins in the blood) in *infancy*.[8] As yet unresolved is the role that vaccines given in infancy play in producing this immunologic disorder. However, for many years immunologists have been aware of a state of anergy (immunologic unresponsiveness) following vaccination. J. A. Brody and others reported that live-virus vaccines have been shown to transiently suppress tuberculin sensitivity.[9, 10]

As reviewed in the booklet *The Dangers of Immunization*,[11] a partial list of vaccine-related diseases and/or immunologic disorders reported in the medical literature would include the following: sudden infant death syndrome (SIDS), Guillain-Barré syndrome, lupus erythematosus, multiple sclerosis, arthritis (in adults following rubella vaccine), and worsening of allergies (in elderly persons following influenza vaccinations).

One of the most extensively documented reports of the indirect effects of vaccines is found in the book *The Hazards of Immunization*[12] by Sir Graham Wilson, formerly of the Public Health Laboratory Service, England and Wales. Although Wilson was not generally opposed to vaccines, he provided a number of documented historical examples in which vaccination against one disease seemed to provoke another.

The first full recognition and description in modern times of immune malfunction following vaccinations should be ascribed to two Australians, Archie Kalokerinos, MD, and Glen Dettman, PhD, as reported in the book *Every Second Child*.[13] In this book Kalokerinos describes his work as a physician in the 1960s and 1970s among Australian aborigines. In early work with these people, he was appalled by the high infant mortality rate; death rates in some areas had soared to 50 percent.

The Australian aborigines were a unique population. They lacked the natural resistance to many infectious diseases to which Western civilization has been exposed throughout the centuries. Also, the aborigines lived in relative poverty on a diet consisting mostly of highly refined and denatured food products.

Kalokerinos (later joined by Dettman) determined that many of the aboriginal infants suffered from acute ascorbic acid (vitamin C) deficiency. He postulated that a compromised immune resistance, due to both a diet lacking in essential nutrients (especially vitamin C) and the presence of infectious illness, placed many infants in a high-risk state. In many children, the injection of vaccine further challenged an already crippled immune system and was enough to bring on death.

The present report, showing lymphocyte abnormality with AIDS-like changes following tetanus vaccine, provides a theoretical explanation for these deaths. It may also provide a partial explanation for the known increase in allergic disorders in our own contemporary population.

Mucosal Vaccinations

If vaccinations are to be used to attempt to control infectious diseases, both intuition and reason should compel us to seek those methods that most closely simulate natural immunity, methods that can be utilized without crippling the immune system of the body.

Today there is increasing interest in and investigation of the mucosal vaccines, of which oral (Sabin) poliovirus vaccine may be considered an example. However, oral poliovirus vaccines, which consist of live viruses grown in animal tissue cultures, are administered in large numbers. Vaccination with these live viruses can and does cause problems.

The subject of mucosal vaccines was reviewed by P. L. Ogra in 1980 and by John Bienenstock in 1983.[14, 15] In contrast to injected vaccines, which bypass the outer defenses of the body, mucosal vaccines more closely follow the processes of natural immunity. Why is this so?

There are five known classes of immunoglobulins (antibodies which serve as immunologic defenses) in the body: IgM, IgG, IgA, IgE, and IgD. The IgC (gamma globulin) antibodies form the largest quantity in the bloodstream, along with IgM (macroglobulins). In contrast, the IgA (secretory immunoglobulin A) antibodies coat the mucosal surfaces of the body, including the gastrointestinal, respiratory, and genitourinary tracts, where they function as "antiseptic paint."[16, 17, 18] From a conceptual standpoint, the IgA antibodies form the first line of immunologic defense of the body, whereas the IgG and IgM antibodies form the last line of antibody defense.

It is clearly evident that most infectious diseases find their way into the body through the mucosal surfaces (lungs, gastrointestinal tract, and so forth). Consequently, "natural immunity" is largely a mucosal immunity involving the secretory immunoglobulin A (IgA) antibodies. Current research appears to support this concept.[19, 20]

Modern vaccines, with the exception (to some degree) of the oral poliovirus vaccine, are contrary to the principles of natural immunity. They are injected into the body, where they stimulate IgG antibodies (last line of antibody defense) rather than IgA antibodies (first line of immunologic defense).

This concept is borne out experimentally. In a comparison of injected, killed poliovirus vaccine with live, attenuated oral poliovirus vaccine, only the oral vaccine produced protective secretory immunoglobulin (IgA) antibodies against polio on the mucosal surfaces of the body.[21]

We would like to see our country in the vanguard of vaccine research, but we are relatively stagnant in this area, with investigations largely limited to the unphysiologic, injected vaccines. Other countries, in contrast, appear to be making significant advances in new dimensions of vaccine research. Writing in *Fortschritte der Medizin*, W. Falk at the University of Graz in Vienna described the administration of oral pertussis (whooping cough) vaccine to 13,770 newborn infants in 1978, 1979, and 1980 in two pediatric hospitals in Austria.[22] It was reported that oral pertussis vaccine lowered the risk of side effects because toxic components were not taken up by receptors in the infants' gastrointestinal tracts. The oral vaccine was tolerated well. The vaccine could be given within an infant's first few days of life, providing the beginning of protection at the strategic time when the child may be at greatest risk. That it appeared to provide both local and general immunity may be another plus.

Present understanding of the total impact of vaccine programs on the immune system is virtually nonexistent. Until more is known, we believe that the oral (mucosal) vaccines are closer to the processes of natural immunity and, therefore, presumably safer than injected vaccines. We can only ask why we are not pursuing this line of investigation more aggressively.

INAPPARENT INFECTIONS AND NATURAL IMMUNITY

For those who are honestly trying to weigh the pros and cons of vaccines, one fundamental question arises: What are the basic differences between natural immunity and vaccines? Each time we scratch our skin we are inoculated with bacteria. When we inhale cold or flu viruses from a sick person, we experience a form of immunization. We may ask ourselves what can be the harm from vaccines when we are exposed to potentially infectious agents many times in the course of an ordinary day? This question is easily answered. A little analysis, based on scientific findings, will reveal that there are fundamental, perhaps irreconcilable differences between current methods of vaccination and natural immunity.

The first difference is the *quantity* of antigenic stimulation in modern vaccines. In the case of natural immunity, it has been estimated that the frequency of unnoticed infections outnumbers clinical illnesses by at least one hundredfold.[23] Evidence for this is substantiated by the high proportion of adults who have virus-neutralizing substances in their blood serum and the number who, during an epidemic, excrete virus without being ill.

If the immune system is maintained "battle ready" by healthful living, adequate rest, sanitation, and simple and wholesome nutrition, then many diseases will pass as subclinical infections without actual illness, or if there is illness, it will be relatively mild. Under these circumstances, we may assume that small amounts of antigenic (infectious) material break through the outer defenses. This limited penetration is probably sufficient to produce an immune response but not to cause illness or to overwhelm the immune system. *Nature heals "homeopathically" (by small doses). Natural immunity is probably based on the same principle.*

The first difference, then, between current childhood vaccines and natural immunity is in the *quantity* of antigenic material. In the former there is the introduction of massive quantities of antigen into the system; in the latter the quantities are small. The second major difference, as outlined in the previous section, is in the route of introduction into the system. Most unnoticed infections enter through the mucosal surfaces of the body (respiratory tract, gastrointestinal tract, and so forth) and result in mucosal immunity. Most modern vaccines, on the other hand, are injected directly into the bloodstream.

If we are to search for methods of vaccination that more closely simulate the processes of natural immunity, it would appear that we are reduced to one area, that of *mucosal vaccines given in small doses.*

This brings us to the next question. Has there been any research involving this method of vaccination? We are aware of one attempt to study homeopathic smallpox vaccine a number of years ago among a small group of homeopaths, the results of which were never published.[24] Beyond this, we know of none.

We believe there is a great wealth of scientific talent in this country that should be directed toward investigation of mucosal vaccines in very small doses. In our opinion, there is no area of scientific investigation with greater possibilities and greater need.

THE ONE CELL, ONE ANTIBODY RULE

In a healthy person, natural immunity is based on a series of body defenses, much as the defenses of a medieval fortified castle. According to this conceptual model, each level of immunologic defense against invading viruses, bacteria, and so forth acts as a shock absorber, so that the impact of invading microorganisms on the bloodstream may be greatly reduced. In contrast to this principle, most current inoculations inject massive amounts of vaccine directly into the bloodstream, thus bypassing the outer defenses of the body.

By way of illustration, let us assume that a child is born with a total immune capacity of 100 units. According to the *one cell, one antibody* rule, once an immune body (plasma cell or lymphocyte) becomes committed to a given antigen, it becomes incapable of responding to other antigens or challenges.[25, 26, 27] Let us assume that 25 years ago this hypothetical child passed through the so-called usual childhood diseases of former decades (measles, mumps, chickenpox, and so on) with relativly minor and uncomplicated illnesses. Considering the extreme efficiency of natural immunity, we may make an educated guess that permanent immunity to these diseases was gained by utilizing only 3 to 7 percent of the total immune capacity. In the case of the routine childhood vaccines, however, it is likely that a higher percentage becomes committed, perhaps somewhere between 30 and 70 percent. It should be emphasized that *once an immune body becomes committed to a specific antigen, it becomes inert and incapable of responding to other challenges.*

While this concept is largely hypothetical at this time, it is compatible with our present understanding of the immune system. As reviewed in current texts dealing with pediatrics and immunology,[28, 29, 30, 31] the human newborn infant comes into the world with a relatively undeveloped immune system. The lymph nodes are small, the plasma cells are sparse in the bone marrow and lymph nodes, and immunoglobulin synthesis is low. Normally, soon after birth the infant begins to respond to multiple antigenic stimuli from the bacterial florae that rapidly populate his or her skin, respiratory tract, and bowel, as well as microbial and parasitic infections (estimated at one every six weeks until age 12) acquired from the environment.

If the immunologic system is normal, this immunologic experience is reflected in progressive hyperplasia of the lymph follicles and the appearance of plasma cells in lymphoid tissues and bone marrow. Also, there is a gradual increase in immunoglobulin synthesis, with gradually rising blood serum levels until approximately six years of age.

According to this model, the immature system of a newborn infant depends on antigenic stimulation for its development. In this sense, *exposure of the infant to viral and bacterial microorganisms may be necessary for normal development of the immune system*, if such exposures come about in a natural manner. When antigenic stimulation comes about in the form of natural environmental challenges, which filter through a series of natural body defenses, then the immune system is developed, strengthened, and matured in the process. If, on the other hand, the immature immune system is compelled to respond to a series of immunizations that bypass the outer defenses and inject massive antigenic material directly into the body, then the inner immune defense system must divert a large portion of its resources and reserves in responding to this immunologic "shock treatment."

The combined effects of massive, repeated antigenic stimulation from vaccines, which short-circuit the processes of natural immunity and which are given at an extremely vulnerable time of life, cannot help but have adverse effects on the immunologic system of the child, possibly leaving this system crippled in its ability to protect the child throughout life.

In addressing the issues involved in current childhood vaccines (which include tetanus, diphtheria, pertussis, polio, mumps, measles, and rubella), there are some uncertainties that should be acknowledged. First, these vaccines can provide protection from the illness caused by their respective infectious agent, but the percentage of children who will be protected by these vaccines varies with each vaccine. For example, the poliovirus vaccine provides a high percentage of protection, whereas the pertussis vaccine provides a low to moderate percentage. Also, the length of time that the protection persists varies with different vaccines. The protection may be of relatively short duration, as with tetanus toxoid, or simply unknown, as with measles, rubella, mumps, and polio vaccines.

This brings us to the most important question: Are vaccines the only alternative for disease prevention? Much of the success over these killer diseases, ordinarily attributed to the vaccines, has been due to improved general health and sanitation. Nearly 90 percent of the total decline in the death rate of children due to whooping cough, diphtheria, and measles between 1850 and 1940 occurred *before* the introduction of antibiotics and widespread immunizations.[32]

As further evidence that sanitation, rather than vaccinations, has played *the* major role in control of the killer diseases (with the possible exception of polio), we offer the example of smallpox. Most people probably credit the smallpox vaccine with playing the major role in recent eradication of smallpox throughout the world, but let us examine the facts. In the article "Vaccines: A Therapy in Question,"[33] statistics show that less than 10 percent of children in developing countries have received vaccines. With less than 10 percent vaccination participation, mass vaccination programs clearly played no part in smallpox eradication in developing countries. Quite possibly, selective smallpox vaccination in conjunction with quarantine measures did play an important part in the protection of those who might be exposed to smallpox, but mass smallpox vaccination was not necessary for the eradication of smallpox.

There is a strong and growing body of evidence that suggests vaccine programs may be weakening the immune systems of our children and thus may be opening the way for other diseases as a result of immunologic dysfunction.

What can be done? While sanitation and improved general health must remain the keystones for control of infectious diseases, there is urgent need for new emphasis on medical research. If vaccines are to be used, methods should be sought that are more in keeping with the processes of natural immunity.

Since the problem is partly political in nature, we believe that major changes in this situation will not come about as long as vaccine programs remain compulsory. If parents are allowed free choice in accepting or rejecting the vaccines for their children, research will be compelled to move ahead, to the ultimate benefit and welfare of our children. In support of this position, we simply point out that vaccines remain voluntary and *noncompulsory* in England, Ireland, West Germany, Austria, Spain, the Netherlands, and Switzerland. The US should follow these examples. In a free society such as the US, there should be inherent checks and balances in order to allow free choice to the individual in matters that concern his or her personal welfare. Nothing else works quite as well.

NOTES

1. Editorial, *Modern Medicine* (May 1983): 57–62.

2. Personal communication.

3. K. K. Eaton, "Incidence of Allergy—Has It Changed?" *Clinical Allergy* 12 (1982): 107–110.

4. D. J. Atherton, "Breastfeeding and Atopic Eczema," *British Medical Journal* 287 (17 September 1983): 775–776.

5. N. R. Butler and J. Golding, eds., *From Birth to Five: A Study of the Health and Behaviour of Britain's Five Year Olds* (New York: Pergamon, 1986).

6. Harold E. Buttram, *The Dangers of Immunization* (Quakertown, PA: The Humanitarian Society, 1983), 27–28.

7. Martha Eibl et al., "Abnormal T-Lymphocyte Subpopulations in Healthy Subjects after Tetanus Booster Immunization," *New England Journal of Medicine* 310, no. 3 (19 January 1984): 1307–1313.

8. R. L. Siegel, Thomas Issekutz, Jerold Schwaber, Fred Rosen, and Raif Geha, "Deficiency of T-Helper Cells in Transient Hypogamma-globulinemia of Infancy," *New England Journal of Medicine* 305, no. 22 (26 November 1981): 1307–1313.

9. J. A. Brody and R. McAlister, "Depression of Tuberculin Sensitivity Following Measles Vaccination," *American Review of Respiratory Diseases* 90 (1964): 607–611.

10. J. A. Brody, T. Overfield, and L. M. Hammes, "Depression of the Tuberculin Reaction by Viral Vaccines," *New England Journal of Medicine* 271 (1964): 1294–1296.

11. See Note 6, 9–15.

12. Graham Wilson, *The Hazards of Immunization* (New York: Oxford University Press, 1967).

13. Archie Kalokerinos, MD, *Every Second Child* (Melbourne, Australia: Thomas Nelson Limited, 1974). Available from Thomas Nelson Limited, 597 Little Collins St., Melbourne 3000, Australia.

14. P. L. Ogra, "Viral Vaccination Via the Mucosal Routes," *Review of Infectious Diseases* 2, no. 3 (May/June 1980): 352–369.

15. J. Bienenstock et al.,"Regulation of Lymphoblast Traffic and Localization in Mucosal Tissues, with Emphasis on IgA," *Federation Proceedings* 42, no. 15 (December 1983): 3213–3217.

16. W. A. Walker, "Antigen Absorption from the Small Intestine and Gastrointestinal Disease," *Pediatric Clinics of North America* 22, no. 4 (November 1975): 713–746.

17. W. A. Walker and Richard Hong, "Immunology of the Gastrointestinal Tract," *Journal of Pediatrics* 83, no. 4 (October 1973): 517–530.

18. W. A. Walker et al., "Intestinal Uptake of Macromolecules: Studies on the Mechanism by Which Immunization Interferes with Antigen Uptake," *Journal of Immunology* 115 (September 1975): 854–861.

19. See Note 14.

20. See Note 15.

21. See Note 14.

22. W. Falk et al., "The Present and Future of Oral Pertussis Vaccination," *Fortschritte der Medizin* (10 September 1981): 1363–1366.

23. *Maxcy-Rosenaw Preventive Medicine and Public Health*, 10th ed. (New York: Appleton-Century-Crofts, 1973), 117.

24. Harold E. Buttram and John Chriss Hoffman, *Vaccination and Immune Malfunction* (Quakertown, PA: Humanitarian Society, 1983), 44–45.

25. F. M. Burnet, *The Clonal Selection Theory of Acquired Immunity* (New York: Cambridge University Press, 1959).

26. R. W. Dutton et al., "Cell Populations and Cell Proliferation in the In Vitro Response of Normal Mouse Spleen to Heterologous Erythrocytes, Etc.," *Journal of Experimental Medicine* 126 (1967): 443.

27. Elliott Middleton, Charles Reed, and Elliot Ellis, *Allergy: Principles and Practice* (St. Louis, MO: C. V. Mosby Company, 1983), 3–4.

28. Victor Vaughan and R. J. McKay, *Nelson Textbook of Pediatrics* (Philadelphia: W. B. Saunders, Co., 1975), 474–480.

29. C. W. Bierman and David S. Pearlman, *Allergic Diseases of Infancy, Childhood, and Adolescence* (Philadelphia: W. B. Saunders, Co., 1980), 27–35.

30. Richard E. Stiehm and Vincent A. Fulginiti, *Immunologic Disorders of Infants and Children* (Philadelphia: W. B. Saunders, Co.,

1980), 36–51.

31. Joseph A. Bellanti, *Immunology II* (Philadelphia: W. B. Saunders, Co., 1978), 65–77.

32. Statistics presented at the presidential address of the British Association for the Advancement of Sciences by Porter, 1971.

33. "Vaccines: A Therapy in Question," *Therapoeia!* (June 1981): 23.

UNVACCINATED CHILDREN

BY RICHARD MOSKOWITZ

The refusal of significant numbers of parents to vaccinate their children has created a sizable group of people needing very much to be studied and has raised a number of important public health issues. Foremost among them is the fear that a large reservoir of unvaccinated persons could contribute to epidemic outbreaks that might involve vaccinated individuals as well. Equally pressing are the immediate practical questions of how best to protect the unvaccinated persons from disease, how to prevent such outbreaks if possible, and how to treat them effectively if they do occur.

The long-term question that interests me the most is what the general health of this unvaccinated group will be like and what we can deduce from this data concerning how vaccines really act.

I would like to begin by proposing that we use the terms *vaccinated* and *unvaccinated* instead of *immunized* and *unimmunized*, since the basis of the vaccination controversy is the belief of many parents that the vaccines do not produce a true *immunity*, but rather act in some other fashion—or, in my view, that they act *immunosuppressively*.

This may sound like a purely semantic distinction, but in fact it bears directly on the first question raised above. If the vaccines conferred a true immunity, as the natural illnesses do, then the unvaccinated people would pose a risk only to themselves. Children recovering from measles, polio, or whooping cough need never fear getting them again, no matter how often they are reexposed in the future. So the reports of large-scale pertussis outbreaks in the United Kingdom since the vaccine was made optional seem to me a convincing argument against vaccinating *anybody*, even those who desire it, because if the vaccine produces authentic immunity, then this rebound phenomenon should not occur.

Furthermore, we should be skeptical about the "outbreaks" that are reported to have occurred. Pertussis, or whooping cough, is actually rather difficult to diagnose conclusively; it requires special cultures or antibody tests that many laboratories cannot perform and that many doctors, in the presence of suggestive symptoms, rarely take the trouble to order. Conversely, there are other cases of pertussis with typical signs and symptoms but negative cultures and no detectable antibodies. In other words, whooping cough as a clinical *syndrome* need not be associated with the organism *Bordetella pertussis*, against which the vaccine is prepared, or indeed with any microorganism whatsoever.

Reservoirs of people unvaccinated against measles, mumps, or diphtheria, on the other hand, *should* result in periodic outbreaks of these diseases. But again, authentic immunity would ensure that *only* the unvaccinated would fall ill, which has never proved to be the case. All known outbreaks of these diseases in the postvaccine era have included large numbers of vaccinated people as well; and in many instances a large *majority* of the cases had previously been vaccinated, some of them quite recently.

The argument that parents should vaccinate their children to protect society as a whole from epidemics does not make sense. Such epidemics argue rather *against* vaccinating the ones who *were* vaccinated but still came down with the disease as soon as they were exposed to it. Likewise, if we accept partial or temporary immunity— conceding that the vaccines are not that effective, but that we have no other alternative to these rebound epidemics—then are we not simply throwing good lives after bad, rather like acknowledging that our patients are addicted to dangerous drugs, yet fearing to withdraw such drugs or even withhold them from others lest the original error be fully or frankly exposed?

Which brings us to the second question, namely, how to protect your unvaccinated child from an acute outbreak of one of these illnesses in the vicinity. The first priority is clearly to *know the illness*— its signs and symptoms, its natural history and vehicles of dissemination, its prevention and treatment.

Rather than reading this information from a pediatrics text and then passing it along to you, I suggest that you read up on these diseases. Even more importantly, meet with your local pediatrician or primary healthcare provider and plan a course of action. If you cannot immediately find someone whom you can work with or relate to, *keep looking*. Your local support system is too important to be left for the time when you need help in a hurry.

Taking responsibility for not vaccinating is no different from taking responsibility for a homebirth or any other form of alternative health care. It calls not for a substitute for conventional care, but rather a different *relationship* to the healing process and the healthcare system based on personal choice and direct participation. We still need help when our children get sick, and we need to know that this help is available to us.

In the event of an outbreak, a great deal can be done to minimize the risk to those exposed and to treat those who actually fall ill—much of which does not involve chemical drugs or vaccines of questionable safety and effectiveness. The homeopathic method, one such approach, uses minute doses of natural substances to stimulate and enhance the natural defense mechanisms of the host. The homeopathic prevention and treatment of specific acute diseases are discussed in detail in the highly recommended book *Homeopathy in Epidemic Diseases* by Dorothy Shepherd, MD, a prominent English homeopath.[1]

The homeopathic approach to epidemic diseases in general was first employed by Samuel Hahnemann in 1799, during an extensive scarlet fever epidemic in the province of Saxony.[2] After he had treated a dozen or so cases in the usual homeopathic fashion, giving small doses of remedies capable of *producing* similar illnesses experimentally, Hahnemann realized that one remedy helped to cure at least 75 percent of the cases, a second remedy covered another 15 percent or so, and the remaining 10 percent required a variety of different remedies corresponding to the unique features of each case. The principal remedy, which corresponded to the *genus epidemicus* (the main characteristics of the outbreak as a whole), was then given out *prophylactically* to people exposed to the disease and also to patients in the early stages of illness—before the critical point, when other remedies would sometimes be needed, was reached.

The results were quite dramatic. Those so treated either did not get sick at all or suffered much milder illnesses, on the whole, than their compatriots who were not treated or who received the drugs and other heroic measures in standard practice at the time. Hahnemann became justly famous for this exploit; since this time, his method has been used with equal or greater success throughout the world in treating numerous outbreaks of cholera, typhus, smallpox, yellow fever, influenza, and other acute diseases of a similar type. Why it has not been more widely influential in this country is a great mystery, and clearly has to do with the historic decline of homeopathy as a *thought form* until the advent of the alternative health and self-care movement of the past ten years or so.

PERTUSSIS

Whooping cough can be quite a nasty and prolonged illness, even in older children, in whom it is seldom fatal or dangerous. It can certainly threaten life in young infants under one year of age, because of the narrowness of the immature laryngeal opening and its particular vulnerability to obstruction from any inflammation or swelling. It is rarely serious in children older than six, and adults, for some reason, rarely contract the illness at all, even when they are exposed and have never had it before.

The incubation period varies from one to two weeks. The illness often begins quite slowly, with some fever, typical upper respiratory symptoms, and a cough that gradually becomes more and more paroxysmal, until the characteristic spasms appear, often terminating in vomiting or tenacious sputum ejected with great violence. Such a cough may commonly persist for six weeks or even longer, suggesting an autoallergic as well as an infectious origin.

The nosode *Pertussin*, prepared from the sputum of patients with this disease, is the homeopathic remedy generally used for prophylaxis of exposed children (*Pertussin* 30c, one dose daily for two weeks after contact); it can also be given in early stages of illness at four-hour intervals. *Drosera* is the remedy most often used for the illness itself, although other remedies may also be needed. For children with a well-developed cough, *Drosera* 30c or *Pertussin* 30c may be given every four hours, or even more often if necessary. A physician should be consulted if the illness is severe.

Homeopathic remedies are available without prescription, but care should be exercised to obtain them from a manufacturer belonging to the American Association of Homeopathic Pharmacies. This way, you will know that they have been prepared in accordance with the standards of the US Homeopathic Pharmacopoeia.

DIPHTHERIA

Diphtheria is rarely seen today in developed countries, but small outbreaks have occurred in the southwestern US (San Antonio in 1977). The illness is primarily a *poisoning* attributable to the toxin (a highly antigenic protein of high molecular weight) elaborated by the diphtheria bacillus. Diphtheria toxin is the source from which the standard vaccine is prepared (diphtheria "toxoid" is the toxin denatured by heat, alum-precipitated, and preserved with an organomercury compound) and is also the source of the homeopathic remedy, or nosode, *Diphtherinum*, which is commonly used for prophylaxis and for treatment of complicated cases.

Diphtheria begins as a "cold" or sore throat after a very brief incubation period of two or three days. The primary infection is usually in the throat or nasopharynx and quickly becomes apparent with a grayish, ulcerating "pseudomembrane," foul breath, high fever, and marked swelling of the cervical lymph nodes (producing the classic "bull neck" in severe cases). Complications such as heart or kidney failure or esophageal obstruction may follow within a few days; severe cases may be accompanied by difficulty in swallowing or talking due to residual postdiphtheritic paralysis that may require further treatment. *Diphtherinum* 30c or 200c may be given in a daily dose for the first three days following exposure. A physician should be consulted and other remedies used if the illness develops.

TETANUS

Tetanus is essentially a *wound infection* complicated by inoculation of tetanus spores into the wound and germination of these under strict *anaerobic* conditions. The infection itself is relatively minor; like diphtheria (and its close relative botulism), tetanus is largely an *intoxication* produced by a highly antigenic protein, tetanus toxin, against which the standard vaccine is prepared by heat denaturation.

Tetanus does not occur epidemically and cannot be passed from person to person, although conditions associated with wound infections (such as warfare) definitely favor it if the spores are present. The spore-forming organisms live in horse manure and, to a lesser extent, in human manure (chiefly among people who keep horses); but the spores themselves are highly weather-resistant and can survive in the soil for decades. They will germinate only under strict anaerobic conditions—such as a deep, jagged puncture wound with enough tissue damage to get the infection started (the proverbial "rusty nail") or a simple wound infection (a severe burn or an infected umbilical cord stump in a newborn) that consumes all the available oxygen and thereby allows the spores to germinate underneath.

Careful attention to wound hygiene will effectively eliminate the possibility of tetanus in the vast majority of puncture wounds. Wounds should be carefully inspected, thoroughly cleaned, surgically debrided of dead tissue (under local anesthesia, if necessary), and not allowed to close until healing is well under way "from below." Two homeopathic remedies that may have a useful role at this stage are *Ledum* 30c, which should be given every two to four hours from the time of the puncture, and *Hypericum* 30c, which should be substituted if any signs of infection are present.

I have had no experience with *Tetanus*, the remedy prepared from the toxin itself, and tetanus toxoid is of no value unless the individual has previously been vaccinated, since a primary antibody response takes at least 14 days, and the incubation period of the disease can be considerably shorter than this (three to 14 days). *Hypericum* can reputedly treat as well as prevent tetanus, but I would recommend giving human antitoxin at the first sign of the disease, since it is far less effective later on.

If you do decide to vaccinate your children with tetanus toxoid alone, there is no need to vaccinate until the child is old enough to walk around and navigate on his or her own (18 to 24 months), at which time the vaccine is far less likely to cause complications.

POLIOMYELITIS

The poliovirus produces no illness at all in over 90 percent of those exposed to it; among others, it causes, at most, an ordinary flu syndrome with fever, weakness, gastrointestinal symptoms, aches, and pains. Even in epidemic conditions, poliomyelitis (the severe central nervous system complication) develops only in relatively few anatomically susceptible persons, most of whom eventually recover.

The typical symptoms of poliomyelitis include extreme sensitivity to touch, irritability, stiff neck, and fine tremors in the early or preparalytic stage, which may look rather like a viral meningitis. Not infrequently, the fever will return to normal for a few days just prior to the onset of these central nervous system symptoms, at which time it will rise again, producing the "dromedary," or double-hump, fever chart. Paralysis—due to inflammation of the anterior horn cells, or motor nuclei of the spinal cord—often appears suddenly and early in the course of the illness as complete loss of voluntary movement in a single limb, or perhaps of the palate and throat muscles (in the dangerous brain-stem or bulbar type), producing disturbances of swallowing. Most of these cases will still recover, with residual paralysis or death often supervening much later, after the acute inflammation has subsided.

The homeopathic remedy *Lathyrus sativus* has been found to correspond most closely in its symptomatology to central nervous system polio, and it has been used with great effectiveness both for prophylaxis of exposed individuals and for treatment in the early stages of the illness, before irreversible damage has occurred. According to Shepherd, a physician named Taylor Smith of Johannesburg used *Lathyrus* 30c, one dose every 16 days, in 82 healthy people (aged six months to 20 years) living in a seriously infected area, 12 of whom were direct contacts. This regimen was continued for the duration of the outbreak, and not one of these people developed poliomyelitis.

Smith also used *Lathyrus* 30c in three doses, 30 minutes apart, for a second group of 34 children who were ill with fever, neck rigidity, and muscle tenderness of varying severity. All of these children recovered promptly and completely, without any sequelae.

Dr. Grimmer of Chicago, a well-known homeopath of the 1930s and 1940s, recommended *Lathyrus* 30c or 200c in a single dose repeated every three weeks for the duration of the epidemic and stated most emphatically, from his own experience, that paralysis will *not* develop in those so treated. Other remedies may be required for the illness itself, at the first sign of which a physician should, of course, be consulted.

Measles

Wild-type measles is a strong, febrile illness lasting at least one or two weeks, with a long incubation period of 14 to 21 days; a characteristically smooth, confluent rash; "measly" or runny catarrh of eyes and nose; and a sizable risk of further developments such as pneumonia, otitis media, or even laryngitis of the croupy or whooping cough type. The incidence of measles in susceptible contacts approaches 100 percent, and in populations not previously exposed to it, the fatality rate may be 20 percent or more. After generations of contact with European and North American cultures, it became a largely self-limited illness for these populations, one still memorable but producing complete recovery and a permanent or lifelong immunity in the vast majority of cases.

The prophylaxis and treatment of measles varies somewhat from outbreak to outbreak, the *genus epidemicus* corresponding most closely to *Pulsatilla* in Hahnemann's series, *Bryonia* in Shepherd's experience, and probably other remedies in other times and places. In the US, largely because of mass vaccination programs, acute measles is now predominantly a disease of adolescents and young adults, undoubtedly involving some genetic interaction with the vaccine virus; it will probably call for still other remedies. *Pulsatilla* remains the remedy most often recommended for prophylaxis, although my own experience is still too limited to confirm or refute it.

Mumps

Mumps, or epidemic parotitis, resembles measles in its highly contagious nature and its predilection for the older age groups as a result of the vaccine program, but it is milder, as a rule. After an incubation period of three weeks, it begins with fever, runny nose, tenderness around the ears, and swelling of the parotid on one side, spreading to the other in a few days. About 25 percent of boys with mumps show swelling and inflammation of one or both testicles; in girls, the ovaries and breasts are occasionally affected. Residual scarring and atrophy of one testicle is sometimes seen in adolescent boys and young men.

The nosode *Parotidinum*, prepared from the saliva of an infected individual, may be used prophylactically, although *Pilocarpine* 6c is the remedy recommended by Shepherd for both prevention and treatment. I have had no personal experience using remedies with mumps.

Rubella

Rubella, or German measles, is the mildest of all the illnesses for which vaccines are presently required and very often escapes detection entirely. In the adolescent and young adult populations—those presently most likely to develop it—the illness may be somewhat bothersome, with arthritic symptoms more likely; the same symptoms are often encountered after vaccination of these age groups. In children, there is no reason to treat rubella at all, in most cases. Pregnant women, especially those exposed in the first trimester, may be given *Pulsatilla* 6c or 30c every day for 14 days following exposure, or every four hours for fever and acute symptoms. Rubella should be suspected in the event of a mild fever, punctate rash, and swollen or tender lymph nodes behind the ears and neck and around the base of the skull—an area seldom affected in other ailments.

People often ask if it is possible to "vaccinate" homeopathically, to use remedies for the same purpose that the vaccines are normally given. This question addresses not short-term prophylaxis in the event of an acute outbreak, which is discussed above, but routine, long-term protection of the entire population against these diseases.

There is some evidence that remedies can be used in this way. I know of several British veterinarians who use homeopathic rabies nosode in lieu of injections to protect their dogs—with no serious side effects and, as yet, no rabies. But in order to do so, they must give the remedy repeatedly throughout the life of the animal—an approach that would be much less suitable for humans. This brings us back to the concept of trying to permanently eliminate suscepti-bility to specific diseases. Why attempt such an uneconomical fanta-sy, as well as an unnecessary one, since the remedies work so splen-didly well when illness is actually present or threatening?

People also ask whether or not homeopathic treatment can be used in conjunction with vaccines. Homeopathic remedies may be given to mitigate the effect or severity of vaccines, just as they have been used with good effect in cases of vaccine-related illness. Certainly, when vaccines *are* given, I would recommend giving *Ledum* 30c—the basic first-aid remedy for puncture wounds— immediately afterward, in three doses 30 minutes apart; and follow-ing them with either the nosode prepared from the disease or vac-cine itself or *Thuja* 30c, the general "antidote" to all vaccines, in three doses 12 hours apart.

Be aware of the possibility that a strong family history of vaccine reaction may greatly increase the risk of receiving that particular vaccine. Any child whose brother or sister or parent reacted strongly or violently to a vaccine should certainly be excused from receiving it, preferably by obtaining a medical exemption from a physician practicing in that state. Likewise, any child whose sibling or parent previously contracted poliomyelitis, or a severe or complicated case of measles or whooping cough or any of the other diseases listed, should not receive the vaccine prepared against that illness. Other grounds for medical exemption include preexisting epilepsy, central nervous system disorder, or any severe or disabling chronic disease where the risk of serious exacerbation from the vaccine outweighs the more imponderable long-term benefit.

This brings us to the final question of the long-term impact of mass vaccination programs on individual and community health. Since I have expressed my concerns on this score,[3] many people have asked if any research has been done to substantiate them. I can only appreciate the irony in the fact that the *compulsory* feature of these programs is precisely what makes it so conveniently impossible to study them—so much so that parents refusing to vaccinate their children deserve to be congratulated for making such research possible and should, in fact, be recruited when it is ready to be carried out.

Equally noteworthy are the unprecedented breadth and scope of the research that will be required. Nothing less than the total health picture of vaccinated and unvaccinated children, followed over an entire generation, will suffice—a great collective enterprise that not only will be exciting and important in itself, but surely will yield invaluable new models for holistic medical research generally; models that will take us well beyond the outmoded focus on single "disease entities" in which we are still imprisoned today. So, regardless of whether or not you decide to vaccinate, I urge you all to think about a mechanism for how collaborative research of this kind can be conducted and how each of us can play our part in it.

NOTES

1. Dorothy Shepherd, MD, *Homeopathy in Epidemic Diseases* (Rustington, Essex [UK]: Health Sciences Press, 1967). Available from Homeopathic Educational Services, 2124 Kittredge St., Berkeley, CA 94704.

2. Samuel Hahnemann, MD (1755–1843), the discoverer of homeopathy.

3. Richard Moskowitz, "The Case against Immunizations," *Journal of the American Institute of Homeopathy* 76 (7 March 1983). Abridged version published in *Mothering*, no. 31 (Spring 1984).

VACCINATION: A SACRAMENT OF MODERN MEDICINE
ADAPTED FROM A LECTURE GIVEN BY RICHARD MOSKOWITZ

See also "Immunizations: The Other Side," 134, and "Unvaccinated Children," 158, by Moskowitz.

In Western medicine, vaccines have become sacraments of our faith in biotechnology. By that I mean, first, that their efficacy and safety are widely seen as self-evident and needing no further proof; second, that they are given routinely to all children, by force if necessary, in the interest of the public good; and, finally, that they ritually initiate our loyal participation in the medical enterprise as a whole. Vaccines celebrate our right and power as a civilization to manipulate biological processes *ad libitum* (and for profit), without undue concern for or even an explicit concept of the total health of populations about to be subjected to them.

These special privileges give some measure of the reverence accorded to vaccines in what can only be called the religion of modern medicine.[1] Its theology, as practiced in the US and to some extent throughout the developed world, involves glaring inconsistencies, such as minimal standards of vaccine effectiveness, that disregard the total health of the organism; enforcement of compulsory vaccination laws in the absence of any obvious public health emergency; and suspension of the normal rules of scientific inquiry in their honor.

THE MEASLES VACCINE

I would like to begin with a brief history of the measles vaccine, which illustrates many issues pertaining to the other vaccines as well. In its natural state, the measles virus enters the body of a susceptible person through the nose and mouth and incubates silently for about 14 days in the lymphoid tissues of the nasopharynx, the regional lymph nodes, and finally the liver, spleen, bone marrow, and lymphocytes and macrophages of the peripheral blood. The illness known as measles is the process by which the virus is expelled from the blood through the nose and mouth, the same orifices through which it entered. This massive, concerted outpouring of the entire immune system culminates in the targeting of the virus by specific antibodies, and the ability to synthesize them on short notice remains encoded as a permanent "memory" of the experience—a virtual guarantee that people who have recovered from measles will *never* get it again, no matter how many times they are reexposed.

In addition to conferring lifelong immunity against the measles virus, the natural recovery process "primes" the organism to respond promptly and efficiently to other microorganisms in the future. Indeed, the ability to mount a vigorous, acute response to infection deserves recognition as being indispensable to the maturation of a healthy immune system.

Measles is about 20 percent fatal in populations exposed to it for the first time. In the US and many other countries, centuries of adaptation and "herd immunity" have slowly and painfully transformed it into an ordinary childhood disease with nonspecific mechanisms in place to help deal with it effectively. The permanent immunity acquired in recovering from the natural disease thus represents a net gain for the total health of the human race.

"True" or lifelong immunity of this type cannot be ascribed to the measles vaccine. In contrast to the natural disease, the vaccine virus produces no local sensitization at the portal of entry, no incubation, no massive outpouring, and no acute disease. It can elicit long-term antibody production only by surviving in latent form in the lymphocytes and macrophages of the blood. Because the vaccinated individual has no obvious way of getting rid of the virus, the technical feat of antibody synthesis presumably represents, at most, a memory of *chronic infection.*

It makes no sense to claim that vaccines render us "immune" to viruses if in fact they weaken our ability to expel them and force us to harbor them permanently. Indeed, my concern and growing conviction is that such a carrier state tends to compromise our ability to respond to other infections as well. In that sense, vaccines must themselves be regarded as immunosuppressive.

In the US, the laws mandating vaccination against measles were enacted in the early 1960s, when the disease was limited almost entirely to elementary schoolchildren and both deaths and serious complications were at an all-time low. With vaccination rates soon exceeding 95 percent in most states, the incidence of measles throughout the country dropped from the prevaccine era average of more than 400,000 cases annually to less than 5,000 cases in the early 1980s.[2] It looked as though the disease would soon be eliminated.

In the 1980s, however, the almost universal faith in vaccinations began to unravel. Measles started reappearing in even fully vaccinated populations, and public health authorities began grappling with the mysterious phenomenon of "vaccine failure."

In 1984, 27 cases of measles were reported at a high school in Waltham, Massachusetts, where over 98 percent of the students had documentary proof of vaccination.[3] In 1989, an Illinois high school with vaccination records on 99.7 percent of its students reported 69 cases over a three-week period.[4] These reports failed to mention the surprisingly low number of measles cases appearing in unvaccinated students. Still, the published data strongly contradicted official claims of a "reservoir" of the disease among the unvaccinated, a mythology used both then and now to frighten wavering parents into compliance.

The data from various outbreaks indicated a resurgence of the disease mainly in older children and adolescents, groups with the highest rates of serious complications. Health officials dutifully suggested that vaccine-mediated "immunity" was only temporary and wore off with increasing age, leaving children unaffected and as susceptible as before, a hypothesis that became the principal rationale for mandatory revaccination in the 1990s.

Unfortunately, the concept of revaccination had already been abandoned after a 1980 study demonstrated that previously vaccinated children with declining antibody titers responded minimally and for an unacceptably short time to booster doses of the measles vaccine.[5] Further refutation came from a sustained outbreak of 235 cases in Dane County, Wisconsin, over a nine-month period in 1986, of which the vast majority occurred among five to 19 year olds, only 6 percent of whom had not been vaccinated.[6]

To their surprise, the investigators of this outbreak found that "mild measles" (defined as typical rash with minimal fever) was far more prevalent in children who *lacked* vaccine-specific antibodies than it was in either unvaccinated children or those whose vaccinations had "taken" properly. This finding suggested that the vaccine virus was responsible for some inapparent or latent activity that had not been suspected before and did not show up on routine serological investigation.

Despite considerable evidence that the "immunity" conferred by the measles vaccine might not be genuine, very few investigators have dared to consider such a possibility. Quite the contrary, the medical authorities have persuaded many state legislatures to allocate additional funds for tighter enforcement of existing vaccination laws. In some inner cities with high incidence, the vaccination age has been lowered to nine months, recapitulating pre-1979 standards, when millions of children were "inappropriately vaccinated" according to guidelines in force since 1985. Now, as then, absurd vacillations and rigid assumptions are catching millions of innocent children in their web.

At present, the "final solution" to the measles question is revaccination, with medical and public health authorities generously throwing in the mumps and rubella vaccines for good measure. A bill currently before the Ohio legislature, for example, mandates documented proof of MMR (measles-mumps-rubella) revaccination before a child can enter seventh grade.[7] Once again, public compliance is being required with little more justification than that the original dose was a failure and the extra one cannot possibly hurt.

OTHER VACCINES

This generic faith continues to bless the pharmaceutical industry in its endless and immensely profitable quest for new vaccines, which in the present political climate is easily transformed into official authorization for vaccinating almost anyone against anything at any time.

In the late 1980s, a vaccine was introduced against *Hemophilus influenza* type b, in response to scattered outbreaks of meningitis in crowded daycare facilities. At first purely optional for two to four year olds, it soon became compulsory for all infants, including those not in daycare. The vaccine is presently given at or before 18 months of age, mostly along with the DPT before the child's first birthday.

Hepatitis B was primarily a disease of adult IV drug users until it found its way into blood banks and became an institutionalized risk for people receiving transfusions and whole blood products. Developed in the 1970s, the hepatitis B vaccine is now being foisted on the entire population because medical authorities have never figured out how to effectively approach or target the drug subculture. In the past few months, the Centers for Disease Control (CDC) and the American Academy of Pediatrics have decided to mandate hepatitis B vaccination for all newborns.[8] Whether or not the US public, increasingly upset about vaccinations in general, will simply acquiesce in this latest baptism of its newborn children remains to be seen.

The search goes on, inextricably linked to the technology of genetic engineering. The chickenpox vaccine, created in the 1970s but never successfully marketed, lacks only an official justification. Currently in the developmental stages are vaccines against Group A *Streptococcus* as well as viruses associated with the common cold and bronchiolitis, all being bred into the gene pool of mice, rats, baboons, and other experimental animals, with no discernible caution or restraint.[9] Also on the horizon is an AIDS vaccine, monstrous even in principle because the people most in need of it are already seriously immunocompromised. A suppressive vaccine given to everyone would not only increase the odds of developing AIDS for those already at high risk; it would soften up the general population as well.

THE DPT STORY

The DPT (diphtheria-pertussis-tetanus) story remains the major battleground of the vaccine controversy in the US. Thanks to consumer organizations such as Dissatisfied Parents Together (DPT), books such as Harris L. Coulter and Barbara Loe Fisher's *DPT: A Shot in the Dark*, and other grassroots initiatives at the political level, the plight of vaccine-injured children is coming to light.

In 1986, despite intensive lobbying by the American Medical Association (AMA) and other vested interest groups, Congress belatedly enacted the National Childhood Vaccine Injury Act, which requires the Public Health Service (PHS) to investigate all reports of vaccine injury and formulate guidelines for compensation.[10] Unfortunately, with a large part of its budget earmarked for advocating and enforcing compulsory vaccination programs, the PHS and its subsidiary agency, the CDC, can generally be counted on to look the other way. Indeed, the new DPT compensation guidelines rule out all conditions other than a few acute reactions (collapse, anaphylaxis, and brain damage) and the comparatively rare cases of chronic encephalopathy or brain damage appearing within seven days of vaccination.[11]

As the DPT battle continues, the unit cost of the vaccine is skyrocketing, as are the number and size of personal injury awards granted and personal injury claims filed against manufacturers. When parents insist, many pediatricians are now willing to give the DT vaccine alone.

Meanwhile, pertussis itself has made a slight comeback, with the CDC reporting a total of about 10,500 cases in the three-year interval from 1986 through 1988.[12] The demographics, however, remain effectively concealed behind bureaucratic terminology. Of those with "known vaccination status," 63 percent had been "inappropriately immunized," and 34 percent had not been vaccinated at all. Because very few cases appear to have occurred in the "appropriately vaccinated" group, the inference is that the vaccine is nearly 100 percent effective. Only by reading the fine print do we learn that those with "unknown vaccination status" (7,700 cases) comprised more than 70 percent of the total. And only by reading between the lines do we reach the patent conclusion that most, if not all, of the "unknown" group must have been vaccinees with no acceptable documentation.

Yet, at least in official circles, faith reigns supreme. One Philadelphia pediatrician, noting several cases of pertussis in infants less than two months of age, recently advocated that the DPT be given even earlier—"as early in life as possible."[13]

VACCINE-RELATED ILLNESS

Whereas modern medicine seeks to define itself *quantitatively*, as a set of technologies for identifying and controlling key numbers, the task of the healer is essentially *qualitative*, to derive the treatment from the unique energy of each patient. As such, a large body of case material has emerged suggesting that vaccines tend to weaken the immune system of many individuals. In addition to immediate reactions (high fever, aberrant behavior, and others), chronic illness (asthma, eczema, allergies, recurrent otitis media, learning "disabilities," and more) has been linked to several of the vaccines.

This connection is confirmed in some cases by pathological evidence that the nosode, or homeopathic remedy, derived from the vaccine itself, proves useful in treating the illness. In other instances, children are helped by many of the same remedies as would have been useful had they not been affected by the vaccine.[14] In other words, the vaccine connection cannot be proved but only suspected, suggesting that the vaccines often act *nonspecifically* to deepen a child's preexisting chronic disease tendency.

A complete picture of how the vaccines act inside the human body will require controlled scientific investigations into vaccinated and unvaccinated children over a period of many years, based on each child's total health picture over time. Only by making vaccines entirely optional, a status they have in many European countries, is this research possible. Society thus owes a considerable debt of gratitude to those parents who have decided not to vaccinate.

AN ALTERNATIVE THEOLOGY OF HEALING

Lest anyone supposes that religious concepts have no place in medicine, here are three aphorisms of the great 16th-century physician Paracelsus, offering a practical and ecumenical theology that healers of all disciplines can accept and live by without having to ram them down anybody's throat:

The art of healing comes from Nature, not the physician.

Every illness has its own remedy within itself.

A man could not be born alive and healthy were there not already a physician hidden in him.[15]

Taken together, these sayings amount to a summary of most everything the present medical system has left out, namely:

Healing implies wholeness. The verb *to heal* comes from the same Anglo-Saxon root as *whole*. Healing means simply to make whole again. Because it represents a concerted response of the entire organism, it implies a totality, a purely qualitative integration on a deeper level than can be defined by any assemblage of parts or approximated by any quantitative measurement.

All healing is self-healing. As a fundamental property of all living systems, healing is going on all the time and tends to complete itself spontaneously, with or without external assistance. This means that the role of physicians and other healers is essentially to assist and enhance the natural process that is already under way.

Healing applies only to individuals. Healing pertains to individuals in unique here-and-now situations rather than to abstract diseases, principles, or categories. In other words, it is an *art* and can never be reduced to a technique or procedure, however scientific its foundation.

To these principles one could add a fourth, governing the doctor-patient relationship and subsisting as a fundamental political and legal right: *Health, illness, birth, and death are inalienable life experiences belonging wholly to the people undergoing them. Nobody else has the right to manipulate or control them, or any part of the body involved in them, without their explicit request or that of somebody authorized by them to act on their behalf.*

A fifth postulate, from the writings of Lao Tzu, would provide an appropriate bottom-line criterion:

A leader is best when people barely know he exists,
Not so good when people obey him and acclaim him,
Worst when they despise him.
Of a good leader, when his work is done and his aim is
 fulfilled,
The people will say, "We did this ourselves."[16]

NOTES

1. R. Mendelsohn, *Confessions of a Medical Heretic* (Chicago: Contemporary Books, 1979), xiv et seq.

2. J. Cherry, "The New Epidemiology of Measles and Rubella," *Hospital Practice* (July 1980): 49; and L. Markowitz et al., "Patterns of Transmission in Measles Outbreaks in the U.S.," *New England Journal of Medicine* 320, no. 77 (12 January 1989).

3. B. Nkowane et al., *American Journal of Public Health* 77 (1987): 434–438.

4. R. Chen et al., *American Journal of Epidemiology* 129 (1989): 173–182.

5. See Note 2 (Cherry), 52.

6. M. Edmondson et al., "Mild Measles and Secondary Vaccine Failure during a Sustained Outbreak in a Highly Vaccinated Population," *Journal of the American Medical Association* 263 (9 May 1990): 2467–2471.

7. LSC 119 0411-1, Sub. HB 168, Ohio General Assembly (1991–1992).

8. *Boston Globe* (11 June 1991): 1–F.

9. "Medical News and Perspectives," *Journal of the American Medical Association* 262 (20 October 1989): 2055.

10. Vaccine Adverse Event Reporting System (VAERS), Public Health Service (1986).

11. Ibid., "Reportable Events Following Vaccination," table 1.

12. "Pertussis Surveillance: U.S., 1986–1988," *Journal of the American Medical Association* 263 (23 February 1990): 1058–1069.

13. *Family Practice News* (15 November 1990): 6.

14. Documented case studies appearing in the original text will be published in a forthcoming issue of the *Journal of the American Institute of Homeopathy.*

15. P. A. T. B. von Hohenheim, *Selected Writings of Paracelsus*, J. Jacobi, ed., N. Guterman, trans. (New York: Pantheon, 1958), 50, 76.

16. Lao Tzu, *The Way of Life*, W. Bynner, trans. (New York: Perigree Books, 1972), 6.

Adapted, with permission, from a lecture given by Richard Moskowitz, MD, at the Annual Conference of the Society of Homeopaths, in Manchester, UK, September 14, 1991.

THE READERS' DIALOGUE 1979–1997

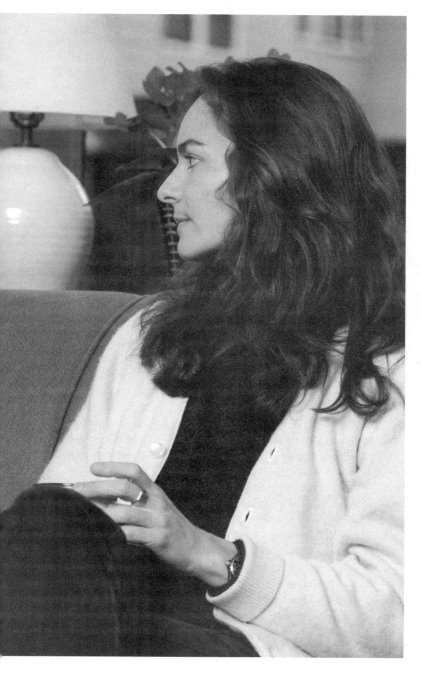

Dear *Mothering,*

Since the birth of our son, Cody (now 19 months), we have tried to make the correct decision about whether or not to immunize. Around two weeks before each shot date, my husband, John, and I discuss it—and then finally decide, yes, it's the right thing for his protection.

Well, when Cody had his MMR shot (at 16 months), his reaction brought an extreme awareness to us. When I signed the consent paper saying I knew that one in a million has a postvaccinal encephalitis reaction, I did not possibly believe that my son would be that *one!*

My little one could not handle the poison from the shot. Ten days after the shot, he was feverish, went into convulsions, was in a stupor, and did not breathe for three minutes! I cannot describe the fear, the panic-state that I was in. My friend Melinda raced us, running stoplights, to the emergency room. I gave Cody mouth-to-mouth resuscitation on the way, which I could barely think how to do. My child was dying. A couple of times his eyes rolled back into his head and then came back out searching my eyes for help. I was so freaked out that I shook his blue, weightless body, pleading, "Please Cody, breathe, breathe . . . come back."

I ran into the emergency room yelling, "This child is not breathing!" Just then Cody gasped and started crying. He turned pink and then pale. He had a temperature of 104° and very swollen glands (the mumps reaction). His fever lasted for 30 hours after that. John and I were by his side, sponging him, holding him, listening for his breath, crying, praying, thankful that he was alive, and wishing the whole thing were over and we had a healthy child again. Three days later he broke out with a measles rash.

It has been a couple of months now since the reaction. I shall never forget it! Not one moment of it.

I have done extensive research lately on the whole immunization business. *Mothering* has been very helpful in providing addresses for information. Eleanor McBean is one author who has very thorough information on the subject.

I now have the whole picture—both sides! I have made my decision not to poison my child again (John agrees). I have a lot of proof to back up my decision, and I'm ready to face any type of feedback . . . and boy does it take courage! I realize that the decision to immunize is totally up to the parents, and I'm not going to be pushy on anyone. I only urge people to find out about both sides before making a decision!

I love your magazine from front to back—every issue. You are inspiring, and you are doing excellent work!

Yours for health and happiness,
Dana Reaves
Fall 1979

Dear American Medical Association,

Simple logic has brought me to a few too many questions concerning vaccinations. There are no answers to be found through the health division; Lester F. Cour, Oregon Immunization Program, to whom I've written previously, has avoided answering my questions specifically.

1) If immunizations do work, if they aren't harmful and they are safe, then why are they repeated? Why aren't they guaranteed, and why were 100,000 DPT serums being located and disposed of?

From Washington, DC (Associated Press): "The government announced the recall Wednesday of more than 100,000 doses of vaccine designed to protect from diphtheria, whooping cough, and tetanus following the deaths of four babies within 24 hours after receiving the vaccine . . ."

The deaths originally appeared to have resulted from the little-understood sudden infant death syndrome (SIDS), also known as crib death.

The government said the Tennessee Health Department noticed a possible connection between one lot of Wyeth vaccine and the sudden deaths of eight infants. But it took no immediate action until it realized early this month that four of the deaths had occurred within 24 hours of a DPT vaccination.

No immediate action was taken "because DPT vaccine is generally administered for the first time at two months of age—precisely the age when the risk of sudden, unexplained death is greatest for infants . . . "

2) Why are adverse reactions kept hush-hush?

3) Why in underdeveloped countries, where immunization programs are used (for example, India), do we still see disease so widespread? This would lead me to think that hygiene, sanitation, and

diet are of utmost importance in preventing disease.

4) If 600 people are unimmunized and six get polio, is this because they were *not* immunized? If 600 people are immunized and six get polio, is this because they were immunized?

I am not sold on the idea that injecting a disease into my healthy son would improve his health.

There is so little anti-immunization literature available. Where is the truth? Somehow, after the swine flu fiasco, I had the feeling I wasn't told the whole truth!

Thank you!
Layah Rutledge
Fall 1979

Dear Editors,

As a pediatrician, I have appreciated *Mothering*'s raising of people's consciousness about many of the things we physicians do "on automatic" in medicine. Minds *can* be opened and stretched.

Because of my training in Western medicine, I am obviously a biased mother, and yet I also agonized over the decision to vaccinate our children. The smallpox vaccination, which was still required when our kids were young, was hardest for me. Finally, the public schools "caught" me and with much fear and trepidation, my children's immunizations were completed in order for them to enter first grade. But I felt somehow deprived of my rights in decision making for my children.

Since then, my family and I have had a unique experience that I would like to share. We moved to a developing area of the world, where my husband and I practiced medicine, and where 80 beautiful breastfed babies would come in yearly to die of tetanus. This was an area where babies who had never had a single canned, frozen, or processed morsel of food would die by droves of whooping cough, and where little children who had never had an antibiotic would suffocate with their diphtheritic membranes. It seemed to us that only the cute little kids got polio. Measles, though, was different; rubella usually killed the sickly.

I am not writing this to frighten readers, but only to say that I would have been much more casual today about immunizations had it not been for the day-to-day reality of living in an area where these diseases are present. You could cite the outbreak of polio among the Amish here, I suppose—they are well known for pure living and contracted polio last August. Or the history of diphtheria epidemics in southern New Mexico—Marie Hughes remembered a village that lost *all* boys under two years of age one year while she was a leader and parents were still frightened of vaccines.

My kids, had they been unimmunized and living in the US, probably wouldn't have gotten these communicable diseases, but not because I am such a good cook of natural foods and rarely use antibiotics. The reason would have been simply that the disease reservoir is low here. That is not to say that breastfeeding, sound nutrition, and the cautious use of medicines aren't all important, too. But we can't lose sight of the real factor: exposure.

We need to give thanks to the generation who went ahead of us and immunized their children so ours may live at a time of little exposure. Do we have a responsibility to future generations to keep the pool of disease down? I think so. As with smallpox, once the pool for any disease gets small enough, then the vaccination will be unnecessary and we will all be winners.

Most parents are concerned about the possibility of dangerous reactions to immunizations, and their concern is legitimate, of course. More development of even safer immunizations can and should be done. We could be a force for insisting that manufacturers of the vaccine for pertussis, for example, continue to refine and improve their product. Why not write to:

Wyeth Laboratories
Professional Services
PO Box 8299
Philadelphia, PA 19101

Lederle Laboratories
Customer Service
7611 Carpenter Freeway
Dallas, TX 75247

Connaught Laboratories
Customer Service
PO Box 187
Swiftwater, PA 18370

and tell them you are not satisfied. Ask if they are devoting research time and money to the improvement of their vaccines. Perhaps, too, a letter to your health departments (local and state) would be effective, as they are the largest purchasers of vaccines. You might also ask why the US pertussis vaccine is different from the World Health Organization recommendations (*New England Journal of Medicine* 303, no. 3, 1980, p. 157).

I think the question of the safety of immunizations is a very important one. But I have lived with and witnessed the danger of not immunizing in today's world.

I suppose, too, I am more deeply concerned about what I see as an even greater threat to children's health these days—a threat against which we cannot immunize. And that is nuclear war. Maybe it is time that we concerned parents move on to tackle what may really ruin our children's lives: an uninhabitable planet.

> *Sue Brown, MD*
> *Albuquerque, New Mexico*
> *Fall 1980*

Dear *Mothering,*

I have a 22-month-old son who will soon be due for his two-year-old checkup. I am advised by my pediatrician that at this checkup my son will have to take a new vaccine called *Hemophilus influenza* type b, or Hib vaccine, to prevent a common cause of bacterial meningitis in children from two to five years old. Any information from *Mothering* or help from other readers on this would be most appreciated. Thank you.

> *Dora Young*
> *Houston, Texas*
> *Spring 1986*

Editor's Note: Although this vaccine is "federally recommended," it is not required.

Hemophilus influenza type b is the leading bacterial cause of meningitis, deep tissue infections, epiglottis, and diseases of the bones and joints. A child's risk of contracting one of these illnesses over the first five years of life is one in 200. Each year one out of 1,000 children are affected, 75 percent of them under the age of two. The current vaccine, however, is not effective in protecting them. It is administered to children at two years of age, although some pediatricians are recommending it at 18 months for children in play group settings. Thus, in the large cultural picture, this vaccine will theoretically prevent 25 percent of the H flu disease.

The risks from the vaccine are, so far, reportedly low. Mild fevers and local reactions have been documented, with less than 1 percent of the recipients registering fevers greater than 101°. The only serious reaction documented has been an allergic response in one child who was then treated without complications.

According to effectiveness studies thus far, of those children who received the vaccine and were included in the study, 90 percent showed protective levels of antibodies.

Dear *Mothering*,

One of the major issues my husband and I have considered is immunizations. After reading all the *Mothering* articles on the subject and sending for the five outside sources advertised, we came to the decision not to have our daughter immunized.

I have strong feelings that it is in the best interest of my child and of future generations not to do this. However, it has never been an easy decision to live with. There are times when I suffer feelings of anxiety and paranoia at the thought of my child contracting one of the serious diseases or viruses. What really *are* the risks of taking your child abroad to countries where these diseases are still present? What about the problem of letting her play with friends who have recently been given the live polio vaccine?

The hardest part is feeling very alone in this decision. None of our friends, so far, has made the same choice. Many were intimidated by the healthcare workers, and now wish they'd been able to give it more thought. Our chiropractor is the only person we know who has given his children no immunizations, trusting in the healthy human body's ability to protect and heal itself.

I would like to appeal to anyone who shares our doubts about vaccines to write to us. Let us know of your thoughts, feelings, information, and experiences. Does anyone know if homeopathic vaccines are in use anywhere today?

Sarah Watson
Suquamish, Washington
Spring 1986

Dear *Mothering,*

I would like to share our family's experience with whooping cough. I am a naturopathic physician, and my wife is an RN. We have a daughter, age six, and a son, age four. Both have had better-than-average health, and neither has received any immunizations.

This fall our son developed a mild fever, which was followed by a cough that gradually worsened. About a week later, our daughter began to cough also. At first I thought that they had a viral bronchitis, and treated them with garlic extract, vitamins, and a dairyless wholesome diet. When the cough became more violent, with spasms occasionally ending in vomiting and sometimes the characteristic "whoop" for air between coughs, I had my son cultured, and our suspicion of pertussis was confirmed.

Public school had just started the day before the lab report came back. We were faced with the likelihood of another four to six weeks of coughing (the typical length of the whooping stage). The public health officer would not allow our daughter to return to school until she had taken antibiotics for five days of a 14-day course to prevent her spreading it. Meanwhile, our daycare provider decided that she could not take the risk of caring for our unimmunized children. Except for a few friends, we felt alone and overwhelmed by the backlash of society's disapproval.

On the bright side, our children were doing fine. Between occasional coughing spasms they appeared and acted completely well. The worst coughing was at night. We agreed to and completed the full course of antibiotics so that our daughter could return to school. As antibiotics do not alter the course of pertussis but only reduce its communicability, we continued alternative therapies, adding the homeopathic *Drosera.* Over the next month, the coughs grew less frequent and severe. Our daughter missed only three days of school. Neither child had any complications or was hospitalized.

In retrospect, Diana and I do not regret our decision not to immunize; we affirm it. Pertussis is a serious disease with potentially serious complications, especially for infants. The pertussis bacteria is prevalent. Immunity from the vaccine lapses after several years, and adults can contract it and mistake it for a cold. The decision not to immunize carries with it a substantial risk of contracting the disease. We are relieved that our children are past it now and have natural immunity. For us, we feel we made the right decision.

The most difficult part of this experience was dealing with the social consequences of not immunizing. We had to put up with the hostility of local pediatricians, who viewed our initial decision as neglect; the disapproval of public health officials; our daughter's loss of her first days of school; and the social ostracism and eventual loss of our daycare provider. The lesson we learned is that we have to be willing to pay the price society extracts for our standing by our convictions.

Brent Mathieu, ND
Billings, Montana
Spring 1986

Dear *Mothering*,

In answer to your letter in *Mothering*, no. 39 (Spring 1986), I'm also getting a lot of questions about the Hib vaccine. One reason why I think I'm receiving so many questions is because people are already suspicious about the old vaccines. Another reason stems from the behavior of physicians who have been taught to use a new remedy as quickly as possible before the side effects become known. Both parents and physicians already know that there is no such thing as a vaccine that has been proven safe and effective. Therefore, the concerns about this new vaccine, designed to protect children against *Hemophilus influenza* infections, meningitis included, are escalating.

I tell parents that when they are faced with the question of whether or not to give their child the Hib vaccine, they should read the prescribing information that the pharmaceutical company has prepared. You will learn that the maximum incidence of *Hemophilus influenza* meningitis occurs before the age of 18 months, whereas the vaccine is only supposed to be given after 24 months of age. You will learn that one shot does not confer enough protection; therefore, the doctors are recommending booster shots. Yet, there is no determination thus far of the need for booster shots or the frequency of the need for booster shots. You will also learn that there are certain diseases caused by the *Hemophilus influenza* germ—such as sinusitis, ear infections, and a variety of others—that are not prevented by vaccine. I therefore recommend against the Hib vaccine.

In addition, this vaccine becomes especially suspect considering that, like every other vaccine, no one has conducted a controlled study on it. That is, no one has taken a group of candidates, given half of them the Hib vaccine, left the other half alone (or given the other half a placebo, like sugar-water), and then compared the outcomes (in terms of both short-term and long-term effectiveness and damage) in the two groups. In the absence of this kind of study, the Hib vaccine remains an "unproven remedy."

Robert S. Mendelsohn, MD
Evanston, Illinois
Summer 1986

Dear *Mothering,*

The most treasured part of my *Mothering* magazines are the letters. Living as I do, amidst another culture in an isolated area of Alaska, I regard the letters as my main chance to communicate with other like-minded mothers. In that spirit, I'd like to share my experience with vaccinations.

When our firstborn (now nearly four) received his first series of vaccinations at two months, my husband and I were only vaguely aware of the possible consequences of the DPT and were surprised at our son's reaction. For at least 12 hours he cried (except when nursing or sleeping), held his body rigid, and gave us no visual recognition. Before the next shot was due, we read a lot about vaccinations and were shocked that the doctor (who was filling in for our regular pediatrician) had given no explanation of known reactions and had never asked us about our family history.

We discussed our concerns with our regular doctor. She said she would give our son the DT (DPT minus the pertussis) as we insisted, but she felt there was no medical reason for this and made a reference to people who worried a lot.

Finally, given what we knew about the possible benefits and risks, and given our remote location—a plane trip away from a doctor or hospital, weather permitting—and the fact that several cases of pertussis had been diagnosed in our region, we decided to get our son vaccinated with DPT again. He is now "up-to-date" with his shots, and aside from mild fever, he has not had another observable reaction.

Still, we worried about what might happen when he received the final booster before starting school. We found a new doctor after our second son was born eight months ago. Before I consented to DPT shots for him, I wanted to find out if this doctor thought our older son's reaction was unusual. He thought the reaction was "neurological" and said he would *not* have taken a chance and given the pertussis to our child again. This information is now part of my son's medical record, and he will never have another pertussis shot.

For the reasons noted above, and because neither we nor our doctor were convinced that siblings necessarily react the same way, we had our younger son immunized with the full DPT series. He's had three inoculations, with no observable reaction.

The lesson for us, and maybe for others, is this: making decisions is much harder than remaining ignorant. Our decision to immunize was an informed one, and we were glad we were able to consider so many factors. Most importantly, we learned to trust our own instincts. Although our oldest son had none of the classic pertussis reactions, such as high-pitched screaming or convulsions, we felt his reactions weren't "normal" either. To think we risked his health three times before finding a doctor who agreed with us is frightening.

Alida Ciampa
Kiana, Alaska
Winter 1989

Dear *Mothering,*

Over the years I have followed with great interest your articles on vaccines. After my firstborn's many bad reactions, I am inclined not to vaccinate my second child. But I am very concerned about the risks. Having conducted a lot of research on the vaccines and diseases, I am still looking for support for my decisions. Are there other parents who would be willing to share their grown children's health histories after choosing *not* to vaccinate?

Jane Stephens
La Conner, Washington
Winter 1989

Dear *Mothering*,

In response to Jane Stephens (Winter 1989), I chose not to have my son immunized, and his health is excellent. He is 11 years old, has never had an ear infection, is rarely sick at all, and is robust and thriving. His health is much better than his cousins' or mine was as a child.

When he was a baby in 1978, I studied the pros and cons of immunization and concluded that my decision could not be based on intellectual thought alone. The literature for immunization is fear-based and does not admit to doubts of efficacy or the possibility of adverse side effects. The literature against immunization is also fear-based, sometimes hysterical. The challenge has been to find the middle way.

After much exploration, I decided to mother my child in ways that bolstered his health and strengthened his immune system naturally, reducing his risk of contracting illness as well as reducing the severity of illness if he were to get, say, whooping cough. Much harder for me to live with would be the consequences of vaccine damage, incurred by voluntarily submitting to an intrusive and questionable procedure. Iatrogenic problems, because they are rooted in ignorance, present a greater threat to me than the conditions they attempt to avoid.

I massage my son and my new four-month-old baby regularly, using Swedish, pressure point, and Reiki styles. We work with breath, visualization, emotional clearing, and Bach flower remedies. We all receive regular chiropractic care. Research has shown that regular massage doubles the levels of antibodies in the immune system. Metabolizing stress goes a long way toward creating and maintaining health. We are aware of the preconditions of illness, and we respond to them by making an effort to regain balance.

Two years ago, against my wishes, my ex-husband had our son, then nine, partially immunized. He had a topical reaction of redness, soreness, and heat at the site of the injection and ran a low fever. Subsequently, he showed symptoms of allergies for the first time ever.

I object deeply to the way vaccines are created—inflicting pain, disease, and degradation on animals. That energy is also present in the vaccines. The possible benefits of vaccination are outweighed by the brutality engendered in their manufacture.

I have never had any problems enrolling my son in preschool or public elementary school because of his not being immunized. I have, on numerous occasions, been severely criticized—by pediatricians and even close friends threatened by the idea that their children's health is not protected unless everyone is immunized. I am sure there are better ways to build immunity to dangerous diseases. Homeopathy is not a legally recognized branch of medicine in Texas, so our family turns to a holistic chiropractor for preventive health maintenance.

The wisdom of introducing potent toxins directly into the bloodstream, where they have easy access to major organs, is questionable. The efficacy of vaccines, using World Health Organization statistics that are controlled for public health measures such as clean water, adequate food, and sewage control, is also questionable. The pedantic rigidity of the medical establishment is well documented, as is the unaccountability of drug manufacturers and individual doctors administering vaccines.

We parents and our children have to live with the consequences of their actions and our own. If we follow our hearts, we can do that, and we can learn from our mistakes. It could be that vaccination is a good alternative to the extensive lifestyle changes demanded by good preventive health habits and stress reduction.

Nancy Klein
Houston, Texas
Spring 1989

Dear *Mothering*,

As a concerned parent, I feel the need to impress on your readers the grave importance of the DPT series of immunizations. I had to deal with the consequences of my son's inability to tolerate the full DPT series when he contracted whooping cough at age 11 months. After three and a half weeks and many doctors, my son's respiratory system had been damaged. He was treated with erythromycin (after he was finally diagnosed), but erythromycin does nothing to the endotoxin produced by the pertussis bacteria, so we spent many sleepless months doing 24-hour respiratory therapy to ensure that our son would live. On several occasions, my son's inability to breathe caused "blue spells" while we could only wait helplessly for the paroxysms to subside. He now has asthma as a direct result of this disease.

Marcie Schonborn
Dallas, Texas
Spring 1989

Dear *Mothering,*

I want to share our experience with whooping cough. I have two daughters, ages three years and five months. We live in a small isolated community of 1,500. Many people here came down with an endless coughing illness; some of them were immunized against pertussis, some were not. None was diagnosed as having pertussis. We found our local health professionals reluctant to test for whooping cough. I insisted, as my children are not immunized. Although I had been immunized as a child, my test was positive.

Even as more people came down with the coughing illness, no tests were done. Because they had been vaccinated against whooping cough, testing requests were refused. One friend who was eight months pregnant went in for a culture; when the doctor determined that she had been immunized, he refused to do the test. She has whooping cough and is due in three weeks.

Among all of our local cases, only a few had the "whoop" sound. We each had our own variation of the cough—all were bad. Some recovered in three weeks, whereas others are still coughing five months later.

My family took no antibiotics. We tried a homeopathic remedy without success. Our best bet seemed to be a good attitude (difficult when surrounded by fear and misinformation) coupled with months of garlic (crushed in a teaspoon with honey), echinacea tinctures, vitamin C, and multivitamins.

Whooping cough taught us temperance and patience. The illness is very long and not much fun to listen to or stay up all night with, but it was not life-threatening for anyone in our community. It's an illness to be avoided, but I'm glad we went through it.

If the disease is detected early enough, a young child can pass through the illness safely. Whooping cough in a healthy person doesn't get that bad. Stress plays an important role. None of us turned blue, not even my infant who has a heart murmur.

A Loving Reader
Spring 1989

Dear *Mothering,*

In all my reading about vaccinations, I have not come across much about tetanus shots. Assuming that vaccinations do work, this is the one shot I would consider for my 14-month-old son, since *Clostridium tetani* are so prevalent in animal feces and soil. Does anyone have references for or personal experience with the disease and the effectiveness of its treatment or prevention by vaccinations? I would also be interested in personal accounts of successful treatment of the other diseases supposedly preventable by vaccinations.

Gabrielle Duebendorfer
Arcata, California
Spring 1989

Dear *Mothering,*

After weeks of researching vaccinations, I've decided not to vaccinate my three-month-old daughter. I'm still undecided, however, about the polio vaccine. What concerns me is the risk of contagion from the vaccine itself. Most children in this country are being vaccinated with the live virus, which is excreted through their bowels for four to six weeks after the vaccine is given.

If an unvaccinated child is around a vaccinated child during these four to six weeks, what is the risk of contagion? Can the adult who changes the diapers carry the virus (from the vaccine)? What about all those dirty diapers? In cotton diapers, does the virus get killed in the wash, or does it go into the sewage system? In single-use diapers, how long does the virus live in the landfills? Are we in danger of its multiplying or seeping into the groundwater? Is this potential grounds for another epidemic, or will we stop administering this vaccine soon (as we did with the smallpox vaccine)?

I realize it would be mostly speculation, but I'm looking for facts, not paranoia. Does anyone know the scoop?

Nathalie Kelly
San Francisco, California
Winter 1990

Dear Nathalie,

While I really do not have "the scoop," I will make a crude

attempt to answer your excellent and thoughtful questions.

There is a risk of unvaccinated children acquiring live polio virus from the vaccinated ones, but it is difficult to quantify. At the very least, it's the perfect rejoinder to those who fear that their vaccinated children are at risk from the unvaccinated ones. There have been a few reported cases of polio in adults, mostly parents of vaccinated children, some severe. Furthermore, the religious fervor for vaccination is such that very little work is being done to assess the risk.

Second, you are quite right that people who change the diapers of vaccinated youngsters should wash their hands, and that the virus undoubtedly does find its way into the sewage (as it did in the celebrated epidemics of the 1950s). Also, the virus might persist in landfills and eventually find its way into the water supply. An epidemic of the vaccine virus (or some vaccine-wild type of hybrid) is also very possible.

Several people have asked me whether the risk of acquiring the virus from vaccinated children constitutes a reason for going ahead and vaccinating. That argument wholly fails to persuade me. The chance of getting the virus from your playmate is doubtless real, but the chance of getting it if you are vaccinated is a certainty!

Richard Moskowitz, MD
Contributing Editor
Jamaica Plain, Massachusetts
Winter 1990

Editor's Note: The American Academy of Pediatrics, in its Report of the Committee on Infectious Diseases (1988), states that "the OPV [oral live polio vaccine] remains in the throat for one to two weeks and in the feces for several weeks, with a maximum excretion time of 60 days. Patients are potentially contagious as long as fecal excretion persists." According to the New Mexico State Department of Epidemiology, the virus is attenuated and potentially contagious only for immunosuppressed individuals.

Dear *Mothering*,

This past year has seen the careful orchestration of the media by public health officials regarding measles "outbreaks" in order to enable them to obtain legislative mandates on second measles vaccination doses ("boosters"), not only for our children but for adults under 33 as well. It is my understanding that ten states have passed postsecondary student vaccination laws for mumps, measles, and rubella. What that amounts to is forced adult vaccination. I heard of no cases of college students opposing the vaccine—partly due to ignorance of the issue, and partly because none of them was willing to give up credit for a class or forfeit a degree.

Public health officials and our legislators were able to push these bills through because there was no substantial public outcry or opposition. I urge *Mothering* supporters to write letters of opposition to the media so that the general public, politicians, and judges can see that there *is* opposition to the vaccination policy.

Bonnie Plumeri Franz
Ogdensburg, New York
Winter 1990

Dear *Mothering*,

I would like to hear from other parents who decided against routine infant vaccination and then did some world travel with their children. What are the physiological implications of later vaccination against diseases that currently exist in other countries?

Dara Wishingrad
Montpelier, Vermont
Winter 1990

Dear *Mothering*,

Long before I became pregnant with my son, I decided not to vaccinate. But after he was born, and after further thought and research, I decided to go ahead with the polio and tetanus vaccines. After his first polio shot at four months, Edward developed a diaper rash that persisted for two full months. He had never had a rash before. He has been fully breastfed, I use cloth diapers, and there has been no change in my diet. No prescribed, over-the-counter, or homeopathic cream has helped.

Now, after his second polio shot and first shot of tetanus, Edward has developed hives. His pediatrician says that this is probably a reaction to the vaccines and that the diaper rash could be as well. He says that these are not reasons to discontinue the shots. But I'm not so sure. What if his next reaction is worse? Much worse?

I would appreciate hearing from anyone who has gone through a similar experience. What did you decide?

Alida Cynric
Madison, Wyoming
Spring 1990

Dear *Mothering*,

After a great deal of agonizing and criticism from others, we have decided not to vaccinate our daughter Chloe. I feel good about this decision and have taken a lot of time to research it. I am worried, however, that she won't be able to contract the normal childhood diseases to develop her own natural immunities. How dangerous would it be if she got these diseases later in adolescence or adulthood? Are the consequences more serious? I'd be interested in hearing from anyone with answers to these questions or support for not vaccinating.

Gretchen Annie Wotzold
Tetonia, Idaho
Spring 1990

Dear *Mothering*,

I would like to share my experience in traveling abroad with my nonvaccinated children. I have been living in Japan (where vaccination is suggested but not mandatory) for the past six years, and my two sons were born on Okinawa and in the Tokyo area. While traveling to and from the US, I have never been questioned about the lack of vaccine records in my sons' passports. Because some diseases are more prevalent in countries other than the US (such as cholera in Thailand and malaria in parts of Africa), I prefer to be careful with my family's overall health rather than accept the risks and questionable effectiveness of vaccines against these diseases. While in Kuala Lumpur and Bangkok, we drank only bottled water and ate at reputable restaurants. If necessary, I would accept the risks of disease over the risks of vaccination, or I would choose not to travel to certain disease-prone areas.

It is my understanding that under the WHO (World Health Organization) code, vaccines are not required upon entering countries that have disease-infested areas; however, a traveler may be quarantined for two weeks upon return to his or her country of origin. The quarantine may be as simple as returning home and reporting to a health official any symptoms found within the two-week period. This procedure may hold true for vaccinated as well as non-vaccinated individuals.

Jennifer Anne Schmidt
Kokubunji-shi, Japan
Fall 1990

Dear *Mothering,*

In response to "Vaccine Updates" in Good News (Fall 1990), I want to share with readers the following information from *The Principles and Practice of Infectious Diseases,* a medical reference book edited by Drs. Mandell, Douglas, and Bennett (John Wiley & Sons, 1985).

Regarding measles vaccine: "Properly administered live measles vaccine has been associated with persistence of measles antibody for up to 15 years after vaccination."

Regarding mumps vaccine: "Although the antibody levels produced are lower than after natural infection, satisfactory titers are maintained for at least 10.5 years after vaccination."

Regarding rubella vaccine: "Rubella reinfection some months or years after receipt of rubella vaccine has also been observed . . . in up to 80% of persons who had received rubella vaccine previously and who were subsequently exposed to rubella during an epidemic.

Reinfections have been more common in vaccinees than in those who had natural rubella . . . It was at one time hoped that large numbers of immune people in a community could prevent rubella epidemics from occurring, so-called herd immunity. However, it has been documented that herd immunity does not decrease the spread of rubella. The question has been raised whether the antibody titer years after vaccination will remain high enough to prevent clinical rubella. Only time and continued surveillance will provide an answer to this question, but should antibody titers fall significantly, a booster vaccination could be given if necessary."

Regarding pertussis (whooping cough): "The marked reduction in the number of cases in recent years has been attributed to the availability and widespread use of pertussis vaccines. However, there was a decline in both incidence and mortality before general use of vaccine, suggesting that other factors may also be operating . . . The presently available pertussis vaccines . . . do not confer either complete or permanent immunity . . . Data suggest that although present vaccines are useful, improvements are needed if optimal protection of long duration is to be provided."

Regarding varicella-zoster virus (chickenpox): "Varicella is a relatively mild illness in normal children. There appears to be no urgency to develop a vaccine for universal use . . . Widespread immunization . . . might lead to a change in the epidemiology of the disease so a larger number of older persons might be affected. One of the major objections to a live vaccine is the tendency of the virus to establish a latent infection. We would have to be certain that vaccine virus would not produce zoster more frequently or in a more severe form than the natural disease."

After reading this information one hardly wonders why high school and college students have been getting measles; why some states now require college students to show immunity to measles, mumps, and rubella; and why health officials focusing on measles have enacted what amounts to an adult vaccination law, as well as a two-dose requirement. Will health commissioners soon be telling us that four or five measles "boosters" are not only required but necessary to avoid the by then life-threatening possibility of getting the disease?

As for chickenpox, health officials are currently planning a mass vaccination requirement. In light of the above concerns with the chickenpox vaccine, our job is to organize *now* and let our federal and state legislators know that enough is enough. It is my hope that *Mothering* readers will write letters to the editors of their local newspapers, visit their federal and state legislators, talk to family and friends, and help prevent the passage of a chickenpox vaccine requirement. When lots of voices are heard continuously, lawmakers pay attention.

The researchers' concerns about the chickenpox vaccine reflect what appears to have happened with the measles, mumps, and rubella vaccines; yet, instead of reevaluating immunization policy and possibly even recommending against vaccines, health policy officials are forging ahead with a new one.

Bonnie Plumeri Franz
Ogdensburg, New York
Spring 1991

Dear *Mothering*,

My husband, ten-month-old son, and I have recently moved back to Guatemala to live on our farm. I've been searching for information on the different tropical diseases here—specifically, malaria, typhoid fever, and hepatitis A. We've decided not to give our baby the malaria prophylaxis, Chloroquine, after reading about the risks involved; he has taken it three times and vomited after each dose. He was also extremely sick after one typhoid vaccination, so we've opted against this inoculation, too. As for the hepatitis vaccine, it must be given every four months, which raises a number of questions.

Traditional doctors are in favor of all these medicines, but I would like to know what other families in tropical areas have done.

Sarah Lee
Izabal, Guatemala
Spring 1991

Dear *Mothering*,

The Centers for Disease Control (CDC) has recommended a series of three vaccinations against hepatitis B for all infants and teenagers. Hepatitis B is considered a sexually transmitted disease, affecting especially those who share intravenous drug needles or who have multiple sexual partners. The vaccine will not be voluntary as are other preventive measures for sexual health, such as condom use. Moreover, most children will be vaccinated before reaching an age at which they can make decisions about drug use and sexual activity.

For *infants?* The "experts" say this is the best course to take to ensure that all young people are protected before they become sexually active. I say, "Enough is enough!" Not even exemptions are guaranteed: almost all states have a built-in provision to rescind exemptions in the case of an epidemic declared by health authorities.

The mandating of the hepatitis B vaccine is expected to be taken on in most 1992 legislative sessions, "at the request of the Department of Health." In some states, such as New Mexico, the vaccine will automatically become required because immunization law states that vaccines considered "standard medical practice" should be adopted by the state.

I urge readers to keep this vaccine from becoming law before it is too late. Stand up and take action. Share the information. Write to your state legislators and inform them that you do not want to see the hepatitis B vaccine mandated in 1992, or any other year, and make sure they know you are serious. The CDC recommendation is an inappropriate, unethical, and unacceptable way to handle the problem of hepatitis B infection.

Bonnie Plumeri Franz
Ogdensburg, New York
Spring 1992

Dear *Mothering*,

Thank you for your article "Vaccination: A Sacrament of Modern Medicine," by Richard Moskowitz, MD (Spring 1992). My children's pediatrician tried to discourage me from eliminating pertussis from their round of vaccines. I said, "No, thank you. I grew up with a younger sister who was among the 1 in 365,000 likely to experience a strong adverse reaction to the shot."

My sister is mentally and physically disabled, and battles seizures on a daily basis. In 1958, my father knew her condition was a reaction to the pertussis vaccine. He still remembers the high fever and the vomiting, and recalls vividly how his little daughter, who was "born perfect," cried endlessly the day of her shot. Not until the late 1960s did the mass media come out on the subject, with reports of lawsuits being filed against pharmaceutical companies. Media coverage continues today, although we are not told that the official statistics of risk reflect only "reported" reactions to the vaccine. The American Medical Association (AMA) has been using "cerebral palsy" as a catchall diagnosis to avoid acknowledging the real culprit, and the current trend is to include SIDS as an escape diagnosis.

Your informative articles support my suspicions about the pertussis and other unnecessary, if not harmful, vaccines. My parents would have been thankful for this information 32 years ago, when vaccinations were the "thing to do." We would have gladly traded a shot for a lifetime of watching a loved one struggle from day to day.

I, like many others, await each action-packed issue of *Mothering*. The articles are strong, and the subjects often controversial, leading me to new insights and challenges in my approach to mothering and helping me view other approaches with an open mind. Each issue inspires me to write and get involved, yet never so much as this one did.

Denise Shaffer
Rohnert Park, California
Summer 1992

Dear Dr. Moskowitz,

When I first became a mother, I was afraid to look at some of the issues concerning my baby's health. Due to my ignorance and fear of "knowing too much" (a phrase used by one of my obstetricians), I allowed my daughter to be vaccinated several times. Then I sent away for *Mothering*'s booklet *Vaccinations*. After reading it and talking with mothers who had opted not to have their children vaccinated, I decided against further inoculations.

The last vaccination my daughter received was the MMR vaccine, at 16 months of age. Prior to that, she had three DPT shots, resulting in fever, lumps at the vaccination site, and personality changes lasting about three days. I myself have multiple allergies—which I now know is a contraindication for the DPT vaccine.

My daughter, three years old and still nursing, has demonstrated sensitivities to quite a few foods and environmental substances. She has had one ear infection (we try to avoid dairy products), which we treated with antibiotics. And she always seems to look "lousy." My question is: Now that the damage is done, is there any way to repair it? How does one go about rebuilding the immune system? Is there a way to expel the vaccines?

Every time I read about the dangers of vaccines, I want to cry. What's done is done, however. And as much as I would like to, I can't turn back the clock. Is there an answer?

Renee M. Farina
West Willington, Connecticut
Summer 1992

Dear Renee,

I can assure you that your daughter's condition is not uncommon or serious, and will undoubtedly heal itself in time, even if nothing is done. The process could very possibly be speeded up and made more efficient with the aid of homeopathy and other natural therapies as well as a qualified professional who is well skilled in these methods.

Richard Moskowitz, MD
Watertown, Massachusetts
Summer 1992

Dear *Mothering,*

Before the birth of our first child, my husband and I did a lot of research and decided not to allow our children to be vaccinated. In the 11 years since, we have continued to educate ourselves on the subject, keeping up on the latest vaccine trends and developments. Not once have we come across information that would lead us to question our decision. In fact, we are more adamantly opposed to vaccinations today than we were in the beginning.

We have two wonderfully healthy sons who have never suffered the string of "common" illnesses that medical practitioners regard as normal to childhood. Indeed, I was shocked when a family practitioner recently told me that children today will have an average of three ear infections before their first birthday. This goes far beyond acceptable definitions of the term "epidemic," and yet it is considered normal, as is the implanting of ear tubes.

I am convinced that breastfeeding each of my babies for a full three years has played a major role in their overall good health. And I firmly believe that allowing their immune systems to develop naturally, free of artificially produced antigens, has left their bodies strong and vigorous.

With so much in the news about AIDS, I often wonder if there is a connection between this immune deficiency and the use of vaccines. I would be very interested to know if anyone has researched the effects of HIV on unvaccinated populations. Are individuals infected with HIV more likely to develop AIDS if they were fully vaccinated in their youth? Could it be that toying with the immune system through routine childhood vaccines leaves the system so weakened (or undeveloped) that it is unable to fight off this virus later in life?

For me and my family, far too many questions have not been asked, much less answered, to justify adherence to AMA vaccination guidelines. We have endured criticism for our decision—something far more bearable than the guilt we would suffer were we to vaccinate and find out later just how damaging this practice is. In our hearts, we know we have made the right choice.

Sarah Logan
Waco, Texas
Summer 1992

Dear *Mothering*,

We applaud Lynne McTaggart's "The MMR Vaccine" (Spring 1992). Your magazine's continual effort to question mandatory vaccination is deeply appreciated.

Parental choice in children's health care is a key issue. It should be the right of parents to choose the kind of care they believe is best for their children. Thank you for this reminder.

M. Victor Westberg, Manager
Committees on Publication
The First Church of Christ, Scientist
Boston, Massachusetts
Summer 1992

Dear *Mothering*,

With support from *Mothering*, we decided against vaccinating our two children. And while we have never regretted this decision, I have a nagging question: in the event that an emergency arises and a tetanus "booster" shot is recommended, what is my best approach? I anticipate a scenario of stern lectures and scare tactics from doctors. In a stressful situation such as this, I want to be prepared beforehand with true facts and knowledge.

Have readers experienced this? Information, please.

Maggie Heeger
Madison, Alabama
Fall 1992

Dear Editors,

Thank you for publishing the "other side" of the story in "Vaccination: A Sacrament of Modern Medicine" and "The MMR Vaccine" (Spring 1992). However, I am wondering what advice Dr. Moskowitz or others might have for parents, like ourselves, who did resort to vaccination and are now more fully informed. We cannot *un*vaccinate our children. We based our decision on the recommendation of people we trusted at the time. Now what?

> A. Citron
> Bellingham, Washington
> Fall 1992

Dear *Mothering,*

This is in response to the letter from Ms. Bonnie Plumeri Franz on the subject of universal vaccination against hepatitis B virus (HBV) (Spring 1992).

HBV causes a liver cancer and cirrhosis—a terrible, aggressive, and incurable disease that usually does not develop until many years, even decades, after contact with the virus. More than 300 million people worldwide are chronically infected with HBV, and the overwhelming majority of these people are unaware of their infection. They are unknowingly spreading the virus to their loved ones and others; in fact, HBV is spread most often from mother to child. The initial public health strategy was to vaccinate only those in high-risk groups. However, this policy failed, and the virus has continued to spread. The Centers for Disease Control recommendations are based on projections that predict the spread of the virus throughout our country in the absence of an effective vaccine program.

You cannot predict what risk group your children will choose to belong to, and you cannot safely predict if, and when, you or your children will have an experience with this virus. Dr. Baruch Blumberg, the Nobel Laureate who discovered the virus and developed the original vaccine, estimates that as many as one in three people will eventually become infected with HBV.

At the Hepatitis B Foundation we hear very sad stories from mothers—with no reason to believe they were infected—passing the virus on to their children. One such story in particular motivated me, along with family and friends, to establish the Hepatitis B Foundation.

The current HBV vaccine is the safest vaccine ever made, and there *is* good reason to promote its widespread use. For further information, please contact the Hepatitis B Foundation, Box 464, New Hope, PA 18938; 215-955-7952. Fax: 215-923-7144.

Timothy M. Block, PhD
Associate Professor
Jefferson Cancer Institute
Jefferson Medical College
Fall 1992

Dear Editor,

The National Vaccine Information Center, Dissatisfied Parents Together (NVIC/DPT)—a national, nonprofit organization concerned with vaccine safety—would like to offer information for anyone concerned about childhood vaccines.

As of April 15, 1992, doctors and other healthcare professionals are required by law to provide parents with educational brochures on diseases, vaccines, and the identifying and reporting of serious reactions. These brochures should be read *well* before your child's vaccination appointment so that you can prepare questions for your doctor and familiarize yourself with contraindications for each vaccine, as well as possible side effects. The federal government receives nearly 1,000 reports of adverse reactions to vaccines *each month*. Sadly, vaccine injury and death are very real. Although most children do not suffer serious problems from vaccinations, when vaccine injury happens to your child, the risks are 100 percent.

The most complete source of information on warnings, reactions, and vaccine schedules is the package insert for each vaccine. This information has been compiled by the manufacturer under FDA supervision. The same information may be found in the *Physician's Desk Reference*, available in libraries, doctors' offices, and pharmacies. Use this material to evaluate any vaccine-related information you might be given. For further information and materials, please write: NVIC/DPT 512 W. Maple Avenue, Vienna, VA 22180.

Ann Millan, Director
NVIC/DPT
Vienna, Virginia
Fall 1992

Dear *Mothering,*

I've listened to parents of vaccinated children advocate vaccinations. I've seen extremely healthy unvaccinated children. I know of children who have been severely damaged by vaccines. One piece of the puzzle is missing: do any parents regret their decision to not vaccinate?

Suzette Lucas
Robbinsville, New Jersey
Spring 1993

Dear *Mothering,*

We have not yet vaccinated our son, and are wondering if continued nonvaccination is advisable. We are planning to live in an area of the world where disease is more common than in North America, and where healthcare standards are lower. We have not seen this matter answered in your articles or letters on vaccination, and would appreciate a look at the risks of vaccination—or of not vaccinating—from such a perspective.

Christine Peringer
Clayton, Ontario
Summer 1993

Dear A. Citron (Fall/Winter 1992),

You asked how you could "unvaccinate" your children now that you are more fully informed about the downside of vaccinations. I have a different experience: I chose *not* to give my sons the pertussis vaccine, and last fall they were diagnosed with pertussis syndrome. After some initial coldlike symptoms, they went on to suffer intense spasmodic coughing spells for over two and a half months. Most of these spells led to severe reflex gagging and vomiting as often as ten times a day and several times at night. My younger son coughed with the characteristic whooping sound as he gasped for air.

We tried homeopathic remedies, antibiotics, and conventional cough medicine. None helped. Although my boys gradually got better, I could not help but think that if they had been infants with smaller lungs and less general strength and stamina, this illness may have killed them.

If the question is whether or not to expose one's children to an imperfect vaccine that could hurt them, the answer is plainly no. The harder question is whether to expose them to the vaccine or to a dreadful, conceivably deadly disease. The answer to that question is far less clear and far more individual. Electing to vaccinate a child who tolerates the DPT vaccine may be the right decision for some parents.

Shelley Kramer
San Anselmo, California
Summer 1993

Dear Suzette Lucas (Spring 1993),

Last fall, we had an outbreak of whooping cough on Kauai. The next three months tested our patience, faith, and conviction in non-immunization. All three of our children—ages nine, six, and two—got full-fledged cases of pertussis. They were as ill as they had ever been in their lives. Whooping cough is a nasty disease with an exceptionally long healing time.

Our children were racked by coughing fits that often culminated in vomiting. Throughout it all, my husband and I never regretted our decision not to vaccinate them, even though some children who *were* vaccinated suffered a less severe form of pertussis.

Our children are now as spunky as ever, and have gained new strengths from this illness. We are grateful that they have boosted their natural immunity. We are also grateful to an understanding naturopathic doctor, Julian Scott, whose book *Natural Medicine for Children* was invaluable, and to our openminded "traditional" doctor, who attended to us and other unvaccinated families with respect and who served as mediator between us and the Department of Health.

Vaccination is a charged issue, as we so clearly saw when lines were drawn in our community during the pertussis outbreak. We can only urge parents to research their decision and then go forward with as much faith and trust as they can muster.

Lee Roversi and Chad Deal
Kilauea, Hawaii
Summer 1993

Dear *Mothering,*

Does anyone know about the safety of unvaccinated children who swim in public pools? Do the chemicals that are added to the water protect against transmission of the polio virus from those children who have recently been given the live oral polio vaccine?

Secondly, in light of the Clinton administration's effort to vaccinate every child, a parent's right to choose or reject vaccination for their children may be in danger. Already more pressure is being applied. The state of Virginia has passed a law that requires proof of vaccination for homeschooled children. Greater restrictions will no doubt follow, as others in the public sector jump on the bandwagon.

Unfortunately, no organization currently represents the rights of parents who choose not to vaccinate their children. Most parents keep quiet about this issue for fear of legal intervention. Could *Mothering* become a forum for sharing information, ideas, and action on this topic? We cannot sit back and allow an aggressive vaccination campaign to force us to submit our children to invasive medical procedures that are likely harmful and possibly life threatening.

The time has come to make ourselves heard! Readers, write to President Bill Clinton, your congressional and state representatives, and the opinion/editorial page of your local newspapers. Demand that a parent's right to choose be federally guaranteed.

Shirlee Keller
Woodbridge, Virginia
Fall 1993

Dear *Mothering,*

I am extremely concerned about the Clinton administration's universal vaccine program. I see no indication that the federal government is considering any research that questions the safety and effectiveness of vaccines. Naturally, the Clintons' efforts have the wholehearted support of the medical and pharmaceutical communities that reap billions in profits from compulsory vaccines. We, as concerned parents, must speak out to protect our right to make decisions about vaccines without further government interference.

Deborah S. Werksman
Bridgeport, Connecticut
Fall 1993

Dear *Mothering,*

I had an adverse reaction to a tetanus shot four months ago. Although I received numerous tetanus shots as a child, with no apparent reaction, 12 years had passed since my last booster shot. This time, I chose the plain tetanus toxoid that is preserved with a mercury derivative rather than an aluminum additive.

The day after the shot, I began feeling pain in my joints and stiffness in my calves when I got up in the morning. A rheumatologist told me I had a reactive arthritis, and that it would go away. Blood tests for rheumatoid arthritis were all negative. Has anyone had a similar experience?

Marilyn Lowe
Salem, Oregon
Fall 1993

Dear *Mothering,*

I am enclosing an article from the French newspaper *Le Monde* about a 1992 outbreak of poliomyelitis in the Netherlands, in which 20 people were hospitalized and a four-month-old baby died. None of those who developed polio had been vaccinated.

Does *Mothering* know, or do Dutch readers know, if this outbreak was natural, or due to a vaccine-related virus transmitted through contact with children who had recently been given the live oral polio vaccine?

Fand G. Bourbon
Pintivy, France
Fall 1993

Dear Shirlee Keller (Fall 1993),

Concerning parents' rights to vaccinate their children or to choose not to, Dissatisfied Parents Together (DPT) was founded in 1982 to educate parents about childhood diseases and vaccines and to help prevent vaccine deaths and injuries. DPT was instrumental in the passage of the National Childhood Vaccine Injury Act of 1986, Public Law 99-660, and landmark vaccine safety bills in several states. In 1989, DPT opened the National Vaccine Information Center (NVIC/DPT), at 512 W. Maple Avenue, Suite 206, Vienna, VA 22180; 703-

938-DPT3.

NVIC/DPT represents the needs of vaccine-damaged children and their families, and is working to reform the mass vaccination system. The center supports an educated parent's right to choose not to have a child inoculated with a vaccine the parent considers dangerous to the child's health. NVIC/DPT is a nonprofit, educational organization, and donations support consumer representation and monitoring of these issues.

Joan E. Bee
Leucadia, California
Winter 1994

Dear Marilyn Lowe (Fall 1993),

I had a severe allergic reaction to a tetanus shot in 1983. During the night following the shot, I awoke with strong aching in all my joints. My sternum also ached, and I had difficulty breathing. After hours of agony and many X rays, I was told that my symptoms were psychosomatic!

I explained to the doctor on duty that I was a psychology major, that I would not accept his answer, and that I would not leave until he could tell me what was wrong. Several hours later, he found some recent information that indicated that I was having a rare allergic reaction to the tetanus shot. The diagnosis was later confirmed by a nurse at another hospital.

Now—ten years later—my daughter's pediatrician assures me that there is no evidence indicating that such a reaction could run in families. My mind is not at ease.

Lisa McColl
Tampa, Florida
Winter 1994

Dear *Mothering,*

Your Good News item "Adverse Reactions to the Vaccine Push" (Fall 1993) jeopardizes my respect for your editorial ability and journalistic integrity. The quote by Terence J. Bovill that "there is not a shred of evidence that [vaccination] either prevents or reduces the effects of any disease for which it is intended" is appalling. It completely discredits an otherwise interesting presentation of the possible hazards of immunization. What possessed you to print patently false information reflecting an abysmal ignorance and medieval ear for a thoroughly studied and time-tested method for preventing disease?

It is an uninformed and perhaps paranoid position to characterize vaccination in general as a money-making scheme for physicians and pharmacists (neither of which I am). Continue to investigate and report on faulty procedures or specific vaccines that may be ill-prepared, but please do not discourage parents from using one of the best methods for protecting their children from dangerous diseases.

Jerry Lane
Sycamore, Illinois
Spring 1994

Dear *Mothering,*

I am a doctor of chiropractic and hold an MSc in both physiology and viral oncology, as well as a PhD in nutritional biochemistry. I have extensively researched the issue of vaccination, and it is my judgment that vaccinating against "childhood" diseases is not an appropriate option for a child's well-being.

Presently, no studies are being performed on the long-term consequences of multiple inoculations. What we do know is that in the 20-month period ending July 1992, there were 17,000 adverse reactions, including 2,252 severe injuries and 360 deaths following vaccination. To complicate matters further, the FDA estimates that only 10 percent of all adverse effects of vaccination are reported by physicians.

In response to the question about an unvaccinated child's exposure to polio in a public swimming pool (Fall 1993): a child given the live oral polio vaccine (LOPV) sheds the virus from both the mouth and nose, in the form of sneezing or coughing, as well as from feces, for up to eight weeks postinoculation. While there is a *possibility* of exposure, the *probability* of acquiring the disease in this way is unlikely. As with any virus, polio can only infect a susceptible host— that is, one who has a less than adequate immune system due to such factors as improper diet, nutrient depletion, and emotional stress. The polio virus must be able to enter the bloodstream of the child to cause a polio infection.

It is estimated that even under epidemic conditions, only 15 to 18 percent of the population will acquire the disease. Most of those exposed to polio, including those exposed under epidemic conditions, acquire a subclinical infection—producing immunity, without the actual disease. The bottom line: the chances of a child contracting polio from the vaccine itself are greater than the chances of a child contracting polio from exposure in a swimming pool.

Ronald G. Lanfranchi, DC, PhD
New York, New York
Spring 1994

Dear *Mothering*,

Regarding Fand G. Bourbon's question about the 1992 polio outbreak in the Netherlands (Fall 1993), although it occurred among members of religious groups that generally do not accept vaccination, *some* of those who developed polio did have some history of polio vaccination. The October 16, 1992, *Issue of Morbidity and Mortality Weekly Report* of the Centers for Disease Control and Prevention states that "at present, the risk for acquiring poliomyelitis in the Netherlands is minimal because of the excellent sanitary conditions and the high nationwide coverage for polio vaccination." I suspect that this is also true for France and other Westernized countries. If sanitary conditions are not excellent, then it appears there should be concern, even in Western countries. I suggest that people become concerned about sanitation and waste disposal *before* they get concerned about vaccinations.

To report adverse reactions to vaccination, call the Vaccine Adverse Effect Reporting System at 800-822-7967.

Bonnie Plumeri Franz
Ogdensburg, New York
Spring 1994

Dear *Mothering*,

I, too, am very concerned about the government campaign to vaccinate every child, and very aware that we need some sort of coalition to provide real support as well as medical and legal resources to those of us who have chosen *not* to vaccinate our children. Approached by mothers faced with such a decision, I have searched and found the resources too sparse and often too radically written to be taken seriously. Some mothers have ultimately allowed their children to be vaccinated because they were unable to come up with a convincing argument in the face of social, medical, and legal pressure to inoculate.

Gina Sylvester
Coatesville, Pennsylvania
Spring 1994

Dear Marilyn Lowe (Fall 1993),

I, too, had an adverse reaction to a tetanus booster shot. When I was 13 years old, I had a mysterious illness, and I discovered only a few years ago that I had received a booster shot several days before becoming ill. Subsequent reading confirmed that my symptoms were similar to those of others who had had adverse reactions to the tetanus vaccine.

I spiked a fever of over 105° F and had swelling and stiffness in my joints. I was admitted to the hospital, and quarantined until the fever subsided. The day after I was released, all my joints became excruciatingly painful, whereupon I was admitted to a different hospital for a battery of tests—all of which, including one for rheumatoid arthritis, were negative. Despite this, I was labeled as having juvenile rheumatoid arthritis.

Now, as a 30 year old, my joints still ache in damp weather and when I become ill. I have written to our government to demand that a parent's right to choose vaccination be federally guaranteed.

Christine Tetreault
Northborough, Massachusetts
Spring 1994

Dear *Mothering,*

My husband and I plan to start a family soon. I have been tested for, and found nonimmune to, rubella. I do not want to be vaccinated against this because of reported side effects such as arthritis.

Are there any alternatives? What is the risk of contracting rubella during the first trimester of pregnancy?

Noreen Sauls
Ridgefield Park, New Jersey
Spring 1994

Dear *Mothering,*

I feel pretty much alone since I made the decision not to vaccinate my second child. I get no support from my physicians, friends, or family, and am constantly questioned about my unpopular decision.

I have changed pediatricians five times in the hope of finding a doctor who will respect my right as a parent to not vaccinate my children. I am glad to say that I have found a good doctor; even though he doesn't agree with me on vaccinations, he treats me with respect and doesn't lecture me every time I'm in his office. My previous pediatricians and their nurses constantly intimidated and belittled me. Not only were they verbally abusive and condescending, but I could not get accurate information from them. Preoccupied with talking me into vaccinating my children, they would not address my concerns about my daughter's possible exposure to the polio virus by coming into contact with recently vaccinated children.

I am reading my 11th book on the vaccination controversy, and can find no middle ground. Information is hard to come by unless you dig deep, and I really do need some advice. How careful should we be with our unvaccinated children in public places? What about shopping carts (so many babies chew and handle the bars)? Should I wait until my daughter is potty-trained before sending her to daycare, where caregivers change lots of vaccinated babies' diapers? Does anybody know the long-term effects of multiple vaccinations on the immune system?

Jo Giampolo
Orange County, California
Fall 1994

Dear *Mothering,*

I have rejected vaccines in general; however, I still have a question about tetanus. We raise and train horses, and know that horses may carry tetanus in their intestinal tracts. What are the risks of getting tetanus from horse manure? What is the proper way to care for puncture wounds? How many tetanus shots does a child need initially? And how important are booster shots?

Vivian Johnston
Oakville, Washington
Fall 1994

Dear *Mothering*,

I am researching vaccinations and would like to hear from readers whose children had either short-term reactions or long-term effects from the shots. Short-term effects may include excessive sleepiness, high-pitched screaming, prolonged crying, limpness, high fevers, blinking or staring spells, paralysis, and seizures. By "long-term effects," I refer to hyperactivity, attention deficit disorder, aggressiveness, learning disabilities, epilepsy, autism, dyslexia, and mental retardation. I would also like to hear from parents whose babies may have died from sudden infant death syndrome, and who think this may be attributed to a vaccination.

If your children are not vaccinated, have they caught any of the childhood diseases? Did they get these diseases if they *were* vaccinated?

René Reeves
Toledo, Oregon
Winter 1994

Dear *Mothering*,

I appreciate your articles on natural childbirth, breastfeeding, and particularly vaccinations. I am wondering if anyone has noticed a connection between the recent practice of vaccinating newborns against hepatitis B and the surge in respiratory syncytial virus (RSV) infections and deaths in very young babies. It seems that when an inoculation distracts up to 90 percent of the immune system, a baby could be left extremely vulnerable to infections such as RSV.

Carolyn Young
Tacoma, Washington
Winter 1994

Dear Friends,

I have a ten-year-old daughter whom I chose not to vaccinate, and have always felt at peace with my decision until a recent visit to our homeopathic doctor for her camp physical. Our doctor suggested that it was time my daughter had the MMR vaccine, because if she contracted measles, mumps, or rubella as an adult, these could be life-threatening, and in the case of rubella, could cause birth defects in her baby if she was pregnant at the time.

I am beside myself. This was a settled issue for me. Is there anyone out there who has been pressured by doctors to inoculate their unvaccinated teenagers?

Judy Medeiros
Newton, Massachusetts
Winter 1994

Dear *Mothering,*

My three-year-old daughter recently had her badly damaged spleen removed, and we have been told that she may need to take penicillin twice a day for the next six months or "for life," depending on which doctor we spoke to. We are concerned about the long-term use of antibiotics.

Similarly, we have special concerns about vaccinations. She was given the pneumococcal and Hib vaccines in the hospital. The pneumococcal vaccine protects against bacteria that the spleen ordinarily deals with. Now we are wondering if she should receive all other standard vaccinations because she is more "at risk" than she should be.

Does any reader have a child without a spleen? Do you have a natural and healthful way to raise your child? What did you decide about antibiotics and vaccinations?

Susan Geil
Chicago, Illinois
Winter 1994

Dear Peggy,

Mothering is a valuable publication that has aided my growth and understanding as a new parent. I differ, however, with your determined stand against childhood vaccinations in the interest of protecting a child: from adverse reactions to a vaccine. Unfortunately, there is a rarely mentioned consequence to the choice not to vaccinate a child: the increased risk to society at large by allowing these diseases to regain a foothold and reproduce within the unvaccinated population. One way this can happen is by exposing children to a historically deadly disease at a time when they might not be able to fight off its effects.

A safe example is illustrated by a recent newspaper article about a 21-day-old boy who, too young to have been vaccinated, died from whooping cough. He contracted the illness via exposure to an older child or adult who carried the bacteria.

My husband and I feel a real obligation to society to vaccinate our child. We urge *Mothering* readers who have chosen not to vaccinate their children to once again consider their desisions in the context of the benefit or loss to society.

Diana M. Hollingsworth
Fayetteville, Arkansas
Winter 1994

Dear Peggy,

As a scientist with four graduate degrees, I would like to respond to Jo Giampolo's questions on vaccinations in the Fall 1994 issue. I have read a dozen texts and over 600 scientific articles on the topic, and I still have many unanswered questions.

How careful should parents be with their unvaccinated children? There are a few basic facts we must consider. Viruses and bacteria are highly opportunistic, and must propagate in nature to escape extinction. To accomplish this, they must try to infect as many people as possible. As hard as these bugs try, only a small portion of the exposed population will develop the actual disease. In the case of polio, Sir McFarland Burnet, a Noble Prize laureate, states that "more than 95 percent of those exposed will develop a subclinical infection" (immunity without disease). In fact, the World Health Organization states that the last case of "wild" polio in the Western Hemisphere occurred in August 1991 in Peru. Therefore, all cases recorded since then have been vaccine induced—by either the vaccine itself or a household contact. *The evidence of association* in developing polio from a vaccine recipient (contact transmission) in 40 reported cases reveals that 30 cases occurred in the vaccinated.

Exposure to the polio virus in a daycare setting is a legitimate concern. Caretakers must take proper hygienic precautions between touching children. The "dose" exposure is more in line with a natural occurrence of the disease, and less with the actual vaccine. There will, however, be a continuous exposure to the virus since most children have been vaccinated. Some parents have exercised the option of administering the inactive polio vaccine (IPV). According to the literature, IPV has not caused a case of paralytic polio to date, yet it does have serious repercussions and has been associated with anaphylactic shock and a blood-clotting disorder known as thrombocytopenia.

Clinical observation and scientific data demonstrate that vaccinations *may* be effective for a portion of the population for an undetermined amount of time and not without consequence. Medical researchers are not yet sure what these consequences are. Some fundamental questions need to be answered: What are the long-term effects of vaccination on the immune system? Is there a correlation between childhood vaccination and the increased incidence of autoimmune diseases such as multiple sclerosis, lupus, and diabetes? How safe are multiple vaccines in infancy? Why are each of the diseases that were disappearing on their own prior to the introduction of the vaccine now lingering, and why are they becoming more indolently aggressive? Are the vaccine manufacturers the tobacco companies of medicine?

Ronald G. Lanfranchi, DC
New York, New York
Winter 1994

Dear *Mothering,*

Thank you for addressing such an important issue as vaccinations (Summer 1996). I was terribly disappointed, however, in your journalistic omissions.

You had a panel intended to answer some very good questions and to provide insight from their respective differing perspectives. This type of format implies that each of the candidates will be given equal time. However, you chose only some of the respondents' answers to some of the questions.

Tell me, for example, why Dr. Moskowitz did not get to comment on the final question? Is this a case of editorial arrogance, ignorance, or journalistic bias? The lack of equality weakens the credibility of your presentation's search for "truth."

Not only was there a lack of equal time in the core article, but the sidebars seemed to emphasize certain perspectives to the exclusion of others. I do not believe that this "special" issue was up to the excellent standards of most of your other issues and articles.

CiCi Reed
La Jolla, California
Fall 1996

Dear *Mothering,*

Where was the other side of the vaccination issue? With maybe the exception of Dr. Moskowitz, no one even presented the "other" side. You conveyed the message to vaccinate—which really exasperates me!

Most of the diseases we vaccinate against are innocuous and self-limited, and not nearly as terrifying as the vaccines' side effects, which were completely underestimated by your panel.

Scientists know very little about the human immune system, and the vaccine philosophy is built only on a theory (Jenner's germ theory). How arrogant of scientists to presume they can improve on something they don't even comprehend. How foolish of us to trust them more than we trust nature—a far superior protector of health! Further, vaccines are not adequately tested before they're injected into babies, and a closer look into the way they are made, shipped, and distributed might shock a lot of people.

No mention was made that vaccines may alter human DNA—a form of genetic engineering with unknown consequences. We are crossing our DNA with that of animals! We are already producing humans with lowered immune systems and creating a society of escalating criminality and violence, cancers, insanity, and behavioral disorders. And what about the hazards of shooting proteins into the bloodstream? How shocking that a few members of your panel actually said that the amount of vaccine (a cocktail) does not affect a child's immunity. How stupid do they think people are?

What happened to the Hippocratic oath, "First, do no harm"?

Daniell Mottale
La Jolla, California
Fall 1996

Dear *Mothering,*

I must commend you on your special vaccination issue. As a chiropractor, I believe in allowing the power that made our son's body to heal and run it without interference. The idea of putting poison into our son's perfectly healthy body is outrageous. We refuse to do something just because it was done to us or because "they" say your child cannot enter school without vaccines. Are those valid enough reasons to do something to violate my son's body? Not in my lifetime!

So thank you for your boldness in facing this major controversial issue and showing both sides of the story. And thanks for your strength, Peggy.

We have recently started a group in New Jersey for parents who choose not to vaccinate. Our quarterly meetings have been left with standing room only, showing us that we are not alone. Interested New Jersey parents can contact us at Parents for Freedom of Choice in New Jersey, 310 Knickerbocker Road, Cresskill, NJ 07626; 201-569-0500

Drew Rubin, DC
Cresskill, New Jersey
Fall 1996

Dear *Mothering,*

I was so grateful that you dedicated your summer issue to vaccinations. As a practicing naturopath, I always tell parents to educate themselves on both sides of the issue, and offer resources and support for either decision. I also warn that both sides are very vested in their beliefs, and that it is hard to get nonhysterical information. Your issue almost struck the balance, but I do have a few concerns and criticisms.

I was disappointed that there was no advice on how to support children's immunity before, during, and after vaccination programs. Supplements and homeopathy have much to offer children who have reactions. I was also disappointed that more natural practitioners were not represented in the "experts" discussion.

In addition, I would like to see you explore the influence of medicine on natural evolution. Evolutionary biology has concentrated on microbes without paying attention to the population with which they interact. The outcomes are dire. In essence, animals, microbes, and viruses evolve together and are interdependent. It is against the survival interests of microbes to annihilate their host. Throughout history, disease has served to strengthen life, culling out the weak and fortifying the immunity of those who survive. Since the advent of modern medicine—including mass vaccinations—we have accelerated the strength of microbes by interfering with their life cycles.

Vaccination ethics extend beyond individuals to their contemporary community. Annihilating microbes and viruses while discouraging natural host immunities from interacting with them naturally may be a dangerous and deadly manipulation of physiology for future generations. Whether or not vaccinations enhance host immunity is not clear.

In the attempt to alleviate suffering, we may have created a greater threat to community and generational health than ever before. As parents, we need to look beyond our individual child's existence when considering our choice in all aspects of life. Otherwise, immune breakdown in allergies, cancer, and AIDS may overwhelm present and future healthcare systems.

Stephanie Georgieff, ND
Orange, California
Fall 1996

Dear *Mothering,*

Regarding the map for state exemption laws for vaccinations prior to school, is it really true that Michigan's Upper and Lower Peninsulas have different sets of vaccination policies? I grew up in the Upper Peninsula and now live in the Lower Peninsula. If your map is wrong, this "Yooper"—one who comes from or lives in the Upper Peninsula—would like to point out your mistake!

Amy Soalberg
Ann Arbor, Michigan
Fall 1996

Editor's Note: Oops. On page 78 of the Summer 1996 issue, the Upper Peninsula should have been shaded gray: medical, religious, philosophical.

Dear *Mothering*,

I commend the staff of *Mothering* on their courage to continually question the established icon of vaccination at a time when this position is especially unpopular. *Mothering* has once again conveyed the important message that parents do have a choice about vaccination, and that this choice should be their constitutional right. The proponents of vaccines, including researchers, pediatricians, public health officials, and politicians—all captured by the drug manufacturers' spell—maintain a war of attrition on accurate vaccine information.

Unfortunately, *Mothering* is not immune to the disinformation campaign about vaccines. The charts and statistics about vaccine reactions reflect the most conservative official vaccine-industry positions. Vaccine manufacturers and their supporters on government panels consistently minimize the true incidence of adverse effects. Their vested interest skews their perspective. Only the most blatant and undeniable adverse events caused by vaccines are officially recognized. The hundreds, or thousands, of specific incidents that occur after a vaccine, the destructive autoimmune responses, and long-term neurologic effects that result in permanent disabilities are ignored and denied in the headlong effort to vaccinate at any cost.

I would plead that parents heed the alarming admonitions of Harris Coulter in his book *A Shot in the Dark: Vaccination, Social Violence and Criminality*, when he states that we are producing a vaccinated population of neurologic cripples. Parents deserve more information, not patronizing reassurance. I encourage them to thoroughly investigate vaccine reactions before making this risk-laden consumer choice for their children.

Randall Neustaedter, OMD, Lac
Palo Alto, California
Winter 1996

Editor's Note: Randall Neustaedter is the author of The Vaccine Guide: Making an Informed Choice *(North Atlantic Books, 1996).*

Dear *Mothering*,

Thank you for your special issue on vaccinations. Once again you show your leadership in tackling an issue that ultimately affects every man, woman, and child.

First, a discussion of vitamins needs to be included in the dialogue. The relationship between vitamin A deficiency and child mortality was noted as early as the 1930s, when supplementation with vitamin A was reported to significantly reduce mortality among measles patients. Research in 1990 again reported the effectiveness of vitamin A supplementation in reducing morbidity and mortality (*JAMA*, 17 February 1993, p. 898). Why has the medical profession ignored that information for more than 60 years?

Vaccine advocates knew as early as 1985 that MMR immunity waned, and they used the "resurgence" of measles, even in vaccinated people, to convince lawmakers to mandate a second dose. It was easier to do this than to admit a possible policy mistake and truly spend time on hearings to reevaluate vaccination policy.

As vaccine immunity wears off—for whatever reason—vaccine advocates are using the law to target us, the "older populations at risk," by changing vaccine policy. Further, with the mandating of the hepatitis B vaccine, immunization policy was quietly changed again to include diseases that are contracted by *behavior*, and in 1995 vaccine policy was expanded to include diseases (chickenpox) that interfere with "convenience and business."

Laws are being changed so that eventually the entire population of the US can be vaccinated when desired. Contrary to the impression by your panel, parents do *not* have a true choice in immunization.

Members of the medical profession push vaccination laws based on bad research, then hide behind these laws as they intimidate parents. Vaccination policy has changed over the last seven years, and in the process, is changing the very nature of our government. What is needed are laws protecting medical freedom of choice.

Unless *Mothering* readers are willing to unite and take action publicly, vaccine advocates will be the ones dictating the immunization laws we live under. Vaccination is not just "the issue of our times," it is a harbinger of the future we leave to our children.

Bonnie Plumeri Franz
Ogdensburg, New York
Winter 1996

Dear *Mothering,*

Your issue on vaccinations was well intended in reporting the "risks and benefits" of vaccinations. However, its general context—that Dr. Moskowitz's expertise represented the "radical"—is dangerous to public health and welfare.

Dr. Montgomery argued the need for future vaccines by saying, "the HIV epidemic has shown how a disease can spread in a susceptible population..." During the 11th International AIDS Conference in Vancouver this summer, new evidence will be presented that HIV-1 and its relative HIV-2 evolved either accidentally or purposefully from cancer virus investigations and vaccine studies conducted in African primates. The near-simultaneous emergence of AIDS in 1978 in New York City and Central Africa is highly suggestive of a common source—most likely, monkey virus-contaminated vaccines tested there years earlier. The issue of monkey virus contamination of the live polio virus vaccines was addressed in *Mothering* only by the "radical" Dr. Moskowitz.

Dr. Gordon's assertion, "Literally thousands of studies have been done showing the efficacy of vaccines. The FDA and similar agencies require these studies prior to approving a new vaccine," is additionally misleading. *The FDA does not assure vaccine safety.* Nor does it even report to the medical scientific community or general public all of the risks inherent in live viral vaccines. Studies that show potential problems, including the contamination of monkey viruses in currently required live polio vaccines, have had little impact on the viral vaccine approval process.

Apparently FDA regulators themselves are denied certain critical information belonging to the vaccine industry. Specifically, FDA regulations are written so as not to compel industry to reveal pertinent information regarding vaccine lots that are not submitted for clinical use but have major ramifications in assessing a vaccine's safety. Moreover, since vaccine development information is considered proprietary, government officials and researchers must shield potential safety issues from public scrutiny.

Leonard G. Horowitz
Center for Complex Infectious Diseases
Rockport, Massachusetts
Winter 1996

Editor's Note: Dr. Horowitz is the author of Emerging Viruses: AIDS and Ebola—Nature, Accident or Genocide? *(Tetrahedron Publishing, 1996).*

Dear *Mothering*,

In your special issue on vaccinations, you did a wonderful job on a difficult and perplexing topic. I am both an attorney and a professional homeopath, primarily working with the rights of individuals to make educated choices in the selection of vaccines.

Your issue did not address the constitutional rights of each and every child and their parents to avoid vaccines solely through the Bill of Rights. The Fifth, Ninth, and Fourteenth Amendments allow for fundamental rights, due process, and, to some degree, freedom of choice. Some will argue that failure to vaccinate causes injury to others—but susceptibility is not the issue, self-preservation is.

I find that vaccinations do not serve to enhance welfare. Rather, they weaken the very fabric of society: our children. Obviously, there are different perspectives on this issue, but ultimately it reaches the level of consequences and effects. Education, and not fear, will eliminate the herding instinct to vaccinate for every harmless disease—especially in the case of vaccines that are no longer necessary.

My new book, *Homeopathic Vibrations: A Guide for Natural Healing* (Sunshine Press, 1996), addresses the vaccination issue, along with some alternative approaches to standard procedures.

David A. Dancu, ND
Boulder, Colorado
Winter 1996

Dear *Mothering*,

Thank you for presenting the issue of immunization to a large and caring audience.

State-sponsored immunization programs are big business, and parents—not the state—should have the final say in whether or not they allow their children to become vaccinated, and to what degree. Childhood inflammatory diseases, such as measles, mumps, and rubella, are "healing crises" and should not be circumvented by immunizations. When worked through and properly treated, these illnesses function as a catharsis to actually strengthen the child's immune system. Much like a muscle that is not used, the immune system can atrophy if never challenged.

With more than 700 children being left in a vegetative state (and more than 65 dying) last year from the measles vaccine alone, one should weigh very carefully mandates such as those imposed by the state. A little-known fact remains that the substrate for more than 90 percent of the world's polio vaccines is made from a kidney cell of the notorious African green monkey. It has long been known that primates harbor viruses dangerous to humans, yet less than one in 100,000 of these serums are tested before they reach their recipients. Are parents allowed or given the opportunity of reading the warning label on the polio serum?

Rodger D. Zill
Charlotte, North Carolina
Winter 1996

Dear *Mothering,*

Thank you, thank you, for covering the vaccination issue. But in the excellent, alarming article "Vaccine Policy" I felt that you left me hanging.

You made an excellent suggestion that we write our politicians about the National Childhood Vaccine Injury Act. However, I'm not savvy or well versed enough to intelligently address my legislators. A sample letter would be helpful. Where can we write to obtain one? Do any readers have a nonsensational letter that I could use as a reference?

Leisa Hammett-Goad
Nashville, Tennessee
Winter 1996

Editor's Note: Author Peggie Cypher notes that the organization NVIC/DPT (listed on page 70 of the Summer 1996 issue) urges parents to register their views on the opinion line at the White House, or to write to Donna Shalala or their congressional representative. NVIC/DPT offers support and education for parents about vaccination. They can be reached at 1-800-909-SHOT.

Dear *Mothering,*

Recent Oklahoma welfare reform laws require all children of recipients of Aid to Families with Dependent Children (AFDC) to be fully vaccinated in order to receive the AFDC grants, unless there is a documented medical reason why these children cannot be vaccinated. There are no religious or philosophical exemptions.

I relied on AFDC for almost two years because I did not receive child support. I am very concerned and angry that, just because a family needs these programs to survive, the state has the right to tell us whether or not we should choose to poison our children with potentially harmful substances.

Andria Bright
Welfare Warriors
Oklahoma City, Oklahoma
Winter 1996

Dear *Mothering,*

In your special issue on vaccinations, Christian Science is listed under "Vaccine and Health-Related Organizations." First Church of Christ, Scientist, Crown Point, Indiana, is one of several thousand worldwide branches of the First Church of Christ, Scientist. It is not a public information resource on the Christian Science Church.

The Christian Science Church takes no public position on social issues, relying on its individual members to inform themselves and to act individually. This includes the issue of vaccination, on which Christian Scientists are under no church dogma to act but are free to make their own decisions. It is correct to state that Christian Scientists deserve an accommodation in public health laws that call for medical vaccination since they have proven that their teaching and practice accomplishes for them what medical vaccination appears to accomplish for the general public.

It is, therefore, neither accurate nor appropriate to include the Church of Christ, Scientist, or Christian Scientists in a list of those who oppose vaccination.

Wade Hardy Jr.
Christian Science Committee on
Publication for Indiana
Indianapolis, Indiana
Winter 1996

Dear *Mothering,*

The vaccine issue was a great gift. Thank you. I learned some things I have not previously come across in my research as a concerned parent. I am already familiar with Dr. Moskowitz's work and writing, and was glad to see the experts' forum include his ideas about the potentially negative short- and long-term effects of vaccines on the immune system. However, I was disappointed that this was not more aggressively addressed in the questionnaire.

Valuable questions include: Are we trading acute illnesses for chronic ones? Why aren't long-term studies, such as 40-year studies, being done? Why haven't more doctors observed or admitted the correlations Dr. Moskowitz thinks are possible? What do we know about the relationship between vaccines and allergies, chronic colds and infections, leukemia, cancer, and immunosuppressive syndromes? And why are these questions constantly skirted in discussions of vaccines and decision-making processes regarding research?

Parents, practitioners, administrators, and researchers serious about the vaccine issue should commit to do what they can to make sure these aspects of the issue are thoroughly addressed. It is possible people will look back on this era in 100 years and say, "What a shame they suffered so much chronic illness when they were only trying to help their children."

Carolyn M. James
San Diego, California
Winter 1996

Dear *Mothering,*

I was very disappointed in the issue on vaccinations. Four of the five "experts" were very provaccination, which is not what I would hope for or expect from *Mothering.*

I was also unhappy with the entire issue being devoted to only one topic. I personally have no interest in reading about vaccinations, having already researched and made my decisions years ago. *Mothering* continues to become more and more mainstream, and I hope this trend will be reversed, though I do understand your desire to reach those who are not at all familiar with alternative parenting issues.

Molly Davis
Maple Valley, Washington
Winter 1996

Dear *Mothering*,

I want to congratulate you for your special issue on vaccinations. I would, however, like to take this opportunity to clarify some of the statements made with respect to the National Vaccine Injury Compensation Program (the program).

As the article mentions, the National Childhood Injury Act (act) of 1986 establishes the program as an alternative mechanism to the tort system for resolving vaccine injury compensation claims. In fact, the program has been greatly successful in meeting its dual objectives: stabilizing a previously perilous vaccine supply and establishing an expedient and effcient forum to provide care for children injured as a result of a reaction to certain childhood vaccines.

As mentioned in the article, the Secretary of Health and Human Services (the secretary) did revise the Vaccine Injury Table to make it consistent with the most current medical and scientific knowledge regarding adverse events associated with covered vaccines. The purpose of these changes, however, was not to narrow the definition of vaccine injury and, in fact, in one instance the definition was expanded to include a previously uncovered adverse event. Rather the secretary was responding to a legislative mandate requiring the secretary to review the scientific literature with respect to the pertussis and rubella vaccines and to revise the table if necessary to make it consistent with current scientific and medical knowledge. In that respect, the secretary entered into a contract with the Institute of Medicine (IOM) to perform this review. The revisions to the table were made based upon that review.

Finally, although the program has been widely viewed as an effective alternative to traditional tort litigation, we need to recognize that it was never designed to be, nor could it ever be, an entirely nonadversarial process. In fact, the act calls for the court to promulgate rules that are "less adversarial, expeditious, and informal ..." We believe that the system is indeed operated in such a fashion.

For more information on the program, your readers may call us toll-free at 800-338-2382 or access our Home Page on the Internet Web site located at http://www.hrsa.dhhs.gov/bhpr/vicp/new.htm.

Thomas E. Balbier Jr.
Director, Division of Vaccine Injury Compensation
Winter 1996

Dear *Mothering*,

Thank you! Thank you! Thank you for your special issue on vaccinations. It came to me at the perfect time, as I have been furiously researching this very issue. The information provided by the medical experts was incredibly helpful and informative.

While I do not think that not vaccinating at all is the best choice, I also do not feel that the childhood vaccine schedule as it now stands is the best choice, either. I have created a vaccine schedule that I feel will protect my son from some of the vaccine-preventable illnesses, while at the same time protecting him from adverse effects that can be caused by vaccines.

Thank you very much for your work in putting together this excellent special issue. You have helped me to make some very difficult decisions.

    Janette Carpenter, RN
    Tucson, Arizona
    Winter 1996

Dear *Mothering*,

Thank you for your vaccination special issue. It truly portrayed all the sides of the vaccination issue and raised genuine, valid concerns.

Five years ago our infant son received his first DPT shot right on schedule. The scariest moment of my life occurred a few hours later, when he turned gray and his breathing became shallow. At the emergency room, we were instructed not to give him the pertussis vaccine again. Thankfully, he suffered no ill effects from his experience.

In light of his brother's experience, I decided not to give the pertussis vaccine to my younger son. A nurse at the doctor's office tried to persuade me to change my mind—to no avail. She did plant doubts, however, which were strengthened as we were leaving, when an infant girl in the waiting room was on her way to the hospital, possibly with pertussis. I wavered all the way home—should I have opted for the pertussis vaccine after all?

Rereading your articles, I stopped my second-guessing and stood behind my choice. I realized that, for me, the worst case scenario was not for my son to catch pertussis—that would be a random happening—but for him to have a serious reaction to the vaccine.

Thank you for helping me make the best possible choice on this issue that has no black and white answers. My choice is not the best for everyone, but it is the best for my family.

Michelle Mewhinney-Angel
Olympia, Washington
Winter 1996

Dear *Mothering*,

There are few magazines I truly devour. *Mothering* remains at the top of my list. You offer information, insight, and support to those of us considered by some to be "alternative," earthy, or just plain different.

Regarding your special issue on vaccination, I strongly believe that the nonvaccination side was poorly represented and incompletely covered. There are many cases, much research, and a wealth of qualified information regarding the issue of unvaccinated children and vaccination reactions. I find it hard to believe that this side of the issue could be fairly and accurately represented with a panel of all MDs. Why not a chiropractor or a member of one of the agencies listed in your references?

Martha R. Herman
Greencastle, Pennsylvania
Winter 1996

Dear *Mothering*,

Your vaccination special issue was terrific! So full of information that is otherwise not widely or easily available to the general public. You confirmed all my decisions so far and gave me just the information I need for the future.

Thanks for an excellent, well-rounded, complete presentation.

Mary-Ellen Vian
Atlanta, Georgia
Winter 1996

Dear *Mothering*,

I read your vaccinations issue with great interest. I have had two very serious reactions to vaccinations. The first was in 1984, when I suffered a cataplexic episode (lost all limb strength and eyesight dimmed) six days after a yellow fever shot. The second was in 1993 when I developed arthritis three weeks after receiving the MMR.

This last condition persisted for ten months. Neither of these instances was reported to the department of health because, according to the doctor, no correlation "could be proven."

I can only wonder how many other adverse reactions to vaccinations go unreported. I am afraid that, despite all of your hard work, this unknown factor renders all of your cited statistics unreliable.

Danielle Lambert
Greenfield, New York
Spring 1997

Dear *Mothering*,

As a mother of three, the main factor influencing my decision to vaccinate was the appalling damage done to my sister-in-law's body by polio during the 1950s' epidemic. However, I remain skeptical of mainstream medicine and keep myself informed on both sides of the issue, carefully choosing which diseases to vaccinate against. I have friends who have chosen not to vaccinate, and I respect their decisions.

A letter published in the last issue of *Mothering* implied that vaccinations were contrary to nature's intention and only serve to weaken the human species. This could be argued for all aspects of modern medicine.

Not to use scientific discoveries may actually be contrary to our "natural role" on this planet. There is a vein of altruism running through the scientific community that is trying to responsibly reduce the mortality rates of our children.

As a society we need to continue debating, questioning, and directing the scientific community in a responsible way. I could not watch my children die from a preventable disease.

Julie Jervis
Cupertino, California
Spring 1997

Dear *Mothering,*

I was disappointed in *Mothering*'s recent vaccination issue. In Peggy O'Mara's introduction, she mentions the "one in 300,000" who reacts adversely to vaccines. Parents should know that this statistic, which is actually 1:310,000, refers to shots, not children. Since children receive up to five boosters of the DPT vaccine, this is a deceptive figure. Parents are often under the impression that because their child apparently survived unscathed from one or more DPT vaccine boosters, subsequent vaccinations will be safe.

Many children, however, have died or been left permanently damaged after repeated vaccinations.

A joint effort by UCLA and the FDA found evidence of high-pitched screaming and death (within 92 hours) following the DPT vaccine. Only reactions occurring within 48 hours, however, were considered significant by the researchers even though the British Encephalopathy Study considered reactions up to three weeks after vaccination as significant.

Only after extensive efforts by the National Vaccine Information Center and Dissatisfied Parents Together did legislation finally pass in 1986 requiring physicians to report adverse vaccine reactions.

Australian researchers have found a correlation between at-risk breathing patterns and the DPT vaccine.

Aside from the issue of toxicity associated with noxious vaccine ingredients, such as formaldehyde, mercury, and aluminum, the use of animal proteins and viruses directly injected into one's bloodstream is seriously questionable. If viral material gains entry to bodily cells and, by nature, joins with the genetic components of the cells, autoimmune responses are inevitable. Indeed, such has been the case with several of the vaccines recorded in the medical literature. These diseases include multiple sclerosis, Parkinson's, Guillain-Barré syndrome, and lupus.

Libby deMartelly
Marlborough, New Hampshire
Spring 1997

Dear *Mothering,*

As a Peace Corps volunteer, I worked in a maternal/infant clinic in a West African village for two years. The mothers in that village taught me invaluable lessons about nurturing infants, and the village opened my eyes to a new understanding of community. It tore me apart to watch the beautiful children of that village die from diseases that could have been prevented by a vaccine. Once every few years, measles would sweep through, taking the lives of the most vulnerable—the babies and the malnourished preschoolers.

Now I am an epidemiologist and the mother of three preschool girls. Like many readers, I am concerned about the risks that vaccines present. I know that my daughters would probably survive the diseases that killed the children of my African friends; my girls are well-fed and have access to good health care. Yet what responsibility would I bear if my child passed the disease to a less privileged neighbor? It's the responsibility of all of us to prevent epidemics. That African village made me see vaccination as part of being a community.

Janet Rich Edwards
Lexington, Massachusetts
Spring 1997

Dear *Mothering*,

As a child I watched a beloved horse die a slow death from tetanus. As an adult social worker, I stood by the bedside of a brain-dead toddler who died from measles complications. My sister has a heart condition caused by an untreated strep infection. My hairdresser's son is mentally retarded, deaf, and legally blind from meningitis at four months.

Yesterday my nextdoor neighbor brought her feverish child outside to play; he had broken out in chickenpox that morning. When I voiced my concern because my children aren't immune to chickenpox, she replied, "All kids have to catch it sometime."

There are no easy answers to the vaccination question. My children are vaccinated because I know that irresponsible parents of contagious children do exist. I don't judge those who choose not to vaccinate, since I understand their concerns. But I do resent parents of any children who do not exercise common sense when exposing others to their children's illnesses.

What I would like to see in the parenting community are more attempts to truly understand another's position on issues like vaccination, circumcision, and education, and less self-righteousness. We need each other.

Kathryn Miller Ridiman
Fort Thomas, Kentucky
Spring 1997

Dear *Mothering*,

Many thanks for your special issue on vaccination, which may well be the first on the subject in a magazine of general distribution. I would like to add a few things and answer a few questions that were not asked.

(Question 4: efficacy of vaccines) My own clinical experience has repeatedly shown that all vaccines also act nonspecifically by promoting relapses in whatever chronic illnesses are already present, if not actually initiating them in the first place. Many dozens of my pediatric patients with recurrent ear infections, sinusitis, asthma, eczema, ADD, etc., have been treated successfully with homeopathy and other natural methods. They remained in good health for many months until their next booster vaccine, which was followed by a complete relapse within two to four weeks. Any vaccine is capable of eliciting this nonspecific response.

(Question 6) The only strategy currently proposed for preventing the resurgence of diseases already vaccinated against is revaccination, despite good pediatric studies showing that booster doses are effective for only a very short time. This well-documented fact effectively refutes the prevailing myth that vaccines confer a genuine but temporary immunity that simply "wears off" after a time, leaving the host magically unaffected by them.

(Question 9) Most parents are intuitively aware of the difference between giving tetanus toxoid and oral polio to a healthy three year old whose immune system is already developing and bombarding newborn infants with a battery of vaccines as their very first immunological challenge. My experience has shown that early and multiple vaccination are both important causes of chronic disease, whereas selective use of a few vaccines as children mature and prove themselves healthy is generally tolerated without serious difficulty. Indeed, because of their general tendency to promote chronic disease, vaccines are most dangerous to children whose immune systems are weakest, often the very population we invoke to justify them. This is why the idea of an AIDS vaccine is monstrous, even in principle.

(Question 14) SIDS, or "crib death," was virtually eliminated when the DPT was postponed until two years of age. In Western Europe, no major increases in reportable diseases occurred when the corresponding vaccines were made optional and available to anybody who wanted them. In Africa, an epidemiologist hired by the World Health Organization in 1985 found that AIDS was most prevalent in precisely those countries targeted in its mass smallpox eradication campaign in the 1970s. In Australia, a SIDS researcher who monitored infant breathing patterns in the late 1980s discovered that normal newborns have occasional brief apnea spells, and that within hours or days of DPT vaccination, such spells are dramatically increased in number, duration, and intensity.

A pertinent question that was not asked is who decides that a particular disease poses such a serious threat to public health as to warrant vaccinating everybody, even against their will? There is zero public discussion of these vitally important matters, as if it were a foregone conclusion that vaccines are so safe and effective, such a net gain for public health, that we simply add on as many as we like without serious risk.

Provaccine representatives from the American Academy of Pediatrics, Centers for Disease Control, FDA, and vaccine manufacturers discuss what disease to target next, what marketing strategy will be required, and how best to mollify a population already vaccinated up to the hilt, not to mention the growing number of primary healthcare physicians who are beginning to realize that enough is enough.

What research needs to be done in the area of vaccination? It turns out that our whole research model is defective, that we consider vaccines to be effective if the incidence of the corresponding acute disease is significantly reduced and large numbers of vaccinated individuals show specific antibodies in their blood. Period. That's all we know and all we want to know.

What such studies fail to answer or even ask is, what is the impact of these vaccines on the individual's total health over long periods of time? Adequate studies will have to include the effect of vaccines on global health and quality of life variables, such as chronic disease patterns, growth and development histories, and common lab parameters, as well as intelligence test scores, school performance, and behavior problems. Ironically, conducting such studies will require large numbers of unvaccinated kids as controls, which is precisely what a policy of compulsory vaccination makes it nearly impossible to do.

In about half the states, the so-called "religious exemption" has been interpreted very narrowly to require membership in certain religious sects that have traditionally opposed medical intervention in general. Vaccine activists in these states would do well to promote legislation similar to that of other states like Massachusetts, where only a deeply held philosophical conviction is required. But even here, the law merely authorizes you to be a "kook," to squawk loudly enough that your rights will be protected, however deviant.

At present, no state gives you the right to make an informed medical decision for your child, to choose this vaccine but not that one, for example. Nationally, then, the most sensible goal would be to make all vaccinations optional, according to the parents' choice, as is now the rule in most civilized countries.

Richard Moskowitz, MD
Watertown, Massachusetts
Spring 1997

Dear *Mothering,*

Some excellent points have been made against vaccination in past issues of *Mothering,* and there's so much more to add. I'd like to point out a few things regarding the letters published in the Spring 1997 issue.

Those who vaccinated their children out of fear of repeating "the horrors of the 1950s," or because they saw someone die of tetanus, measles, or whatever, responded exactly the way the government and the Centers for Disease Control wanted them to: petrified to death and kept as ignorant as possible. Ignorance and fear go hand in hand.

It simply blows my mind to see and hear otherwise educated and intelligent people deliberately looking no further than their own noses. We keep blindly assuming that the "germ theory" works, no matter how many holes it has. Germs are mere precipitators, or triggers, of disease. They alone do not cause you to be sick. The host determines how sick—

if at all—you become when exposed to a germ.

Vaccination is dangerous. It's another of the quick fixes we love so much, but I believe it is a catastrophe waiting to happen. I cannot thank *Mothering* enough for being there, ripping off our blindfolds, and giving us hope of assuming control once again. We do have the power to exert some control over natural disease in children. Once we vaccinate, we kiss that control goodbye.

Danielle Mottale
La Jolla, California
Summer 1997

Dear *Mothering*,

Regarding vaccination, informed consent is crucial. Parents must be given full disclosure of the risks of vaccines, especially particular risks to children who have a history of allergies or neurological problems.

Our daughter, Kaisha, was born with tremors, into a family with a history of severe allergies. When she was a week old, we were told that she might have neurological damage. At two months old, she weighed less than 10 pounds. Nonetheless, the pediatrician told us to vaccinate her, and the public health nurse stated that the only risk from the DTP shot was a fever. We later learned that all of our daughter's symptoms contraindicated vaccination.

Kaisha's legs shook violently immediately after the shot, and she let out a high-pitched scream that lasted 13 hours before she fell into a deep, eight-hour sleep. Chronic diarrhea began two days afterward and lasted for three months. The prolonged high-pitched screaming persisted for five months following the vaccination. A neurologist diagnosed neurological damage with an uncertain prognosis.

Thankfully, we refused more drugs and consulted a homeopathic physician. He helped our baby immeasurably, and the screaming has now virtually gone. Throughout this time I have carried my daughter in a sling night and day. She is developing "normally" and making up for lost time.

I tell my story not to shock or frighten but to encourage parents to get all the information, and to be especially careful with children who are more susceptible to adverse vaccination reactions.

Krista Thompson
De Winton, Alberta, Canada
Summer 1997

Dear *Mothering*,

You were right about vaccination! It is an important and difficult subject of great concern to many parents.

I was more than a little surprised to see a "Special Report" in *Money* magazine (December 1996) about vaccination dangers. This article, "The Lethal Dangers of the Billion-Dollar Vaccine Business," explores the political and financial considerations that shape national vaccination policy. On the personal level, the article cites specific children—and adults—who have been harmed by dangerous vaccines when safer ones were available. Parents are advised to pay extra for the safer forms of the DPT and polio vaccines.

> *Dorothy W. Olson*
> *St. Paul, Minnesota*
> *Summer 1997*

Dear *Mothering*,

I am responding to Dr. Richard Moskowitz's letter in the Spring 1997 issue and specifically his point about parents' being allowed to make an informed medical decision about their child. I agree that if people were truly able to make that informed decision, uniform vaccination would decrease.

I want to vaccinate my children selectively, based on the information I have gathered. My most pressing concern is how I get my children into public school in a state where there is no philosophical exemption. Every doctor I have spoken to has told me that I will have a problem with this. Do you have information that could help me do what I feel is best for my children?

> *Elisabeth Landor*
> *Chicago, Illinois*
> *Summer 1997*

Dear *Mothering*,

I am a registered nurse and am periodically offered hepatitis B shots. I have always turned them down, but I do have a client who is a carrier, and I really don't want to ever get the disease. I need more information on the current wisdom regarding this vaccine and would like to hear others' experiences.

I recently cared for a man who died of a dreadful autoimmune disease that he firmly believed started with a flu shot. No one believed him, but I did!

I am leery of vaccinations that perhaps provide short-term gain but also a long-term loss. It's so sad that our daughters will have no natural immunity to pass on through their breastmilk to their own children!

Julie Deisenroth
Munising, Michigan
Summer 1997

Dear *Mothering*,

I very much enjoy *Mothering*, and am pleased to see advocacy of natural family living and responsive parenting in print. I continue, however, to wonder over the extreme negativity (especially in your readers' letters) toward vaccinations. While parents have responsibility and choice over decisions about their children, this decision seems to have been made into a paranoid "us versus them" battle, with scientists, pediatricians, and public health officials portrayed as a vast, secret government conspiracy.

Let us not return to the Dark Ages in an attempt to maintain natural living. Before vaccinations, millions of people died from now-preventable diseases, no matter how full of vitamins their diets were, whether or not they were breastfed, and regardless of loving nurturing.

Please don't overlook the primary and inescapable reason for vaccinations: they prevent diseases that kill children.

Michelle Ogilvie Hils
Lakewood, Ohio
Summer 1997

Dear *Mothering*,

I would like to know what role long-term breastfeeding plays in the vaccination debate. Are breastfed babies and children less likely to contract childhood diseases? And, if they do develop a disease, are they more likely to recover quickly, with less incidence of complications, including death?

It is my feeling that we underestimate—or intentionally over-look—the impact that breastmilk has on the developing immune system. There is ample evidence on the immunological significance of colostrum and breastmilk. Despite our concern about preventing childhood diseases and strengthening the immune system, the medical profession and society in general are not adamant about promoting breastfeeding as a way to strengthen the immune system.

Do we compensate for this by vaccinating babies at a very young age? What role does pharmaceutical and formula companies' profit play in ignoring the benefits of breastmilk? Why does our society condemn parents who make an informed choice not to vaccinate?

While I do not naively believe that breastfeeding prevents all disease, or that breastfed children cannot experience complications—even death—from childhood diseases, I have the feeling we are not being told the entire truth about vaccines.

Marianne Bataillard
Lacha Biche, Alberta, Canada
Fall 1997

Dear *Mothering,*

I must respond to those readers who think that vaccinating their child is a parent's responsibility to the community.

Our role as good parents is to act in the best interests of our own children, not the public at large. We are not acting as responsible parents if we compromise our child's health for the benefit of the community. It would be a daunting task to make daily decisions based on the consensus of the public (or vice versa). We are not governments; we are individuals trying to do what we think is best for our own child. Choosing not to vaccinate is not irresponsible. Responsibility is keeping your family safe, and this, in turn, keeps us all secure.

If parents feel they are protecting their child by vaccination, then how can they still feel threatened by children who are not vaccinated? How can parents of unvaccinated children be any more to blame for spreading disease than the parents of the many children who acquire an illness despite being vaccinated?

Attacking those who've made the difficult decision not to vaccinate is much more threatening to the real concerns of responsibility, and undermines the need for support of the parental role. This only inhibits a parent's ability to make sound decisions about important personal issues like vaccinations.

Michelle Fletcher
Phoenix, Arizona
Fall 1997

Dear *Mothering,*

I was about to let my long-time subscription to *Mothering* expire, thinking that I didn't need you anymore, when I found out about an outbreak of pertussis just across the state line. Since my children were not vaccinated, I was cautious.

I pulled out a back issue of *Mothering* (Winter 1988) that had an article on pertussis and the experience of Anna Joyce, which guided me to have my daughter tested for the illness, even though our doctor said that it was not necessary, considering her mild cold symptoms and nondescript cough.

She tested positive. We were surprised, yet prepared because of the article. We caught it early: The whole family got on erythromycin and followed the Joyces' course of using homeopathic remedies, as well.

Because I was informed I felt empowered and responsible. Thank you, *Mothering.* Enclosed is my subscription for three more years!

Catharine Scherer
Spokane, Washington
Fall 1997

GOOD NEWS

1987–1997

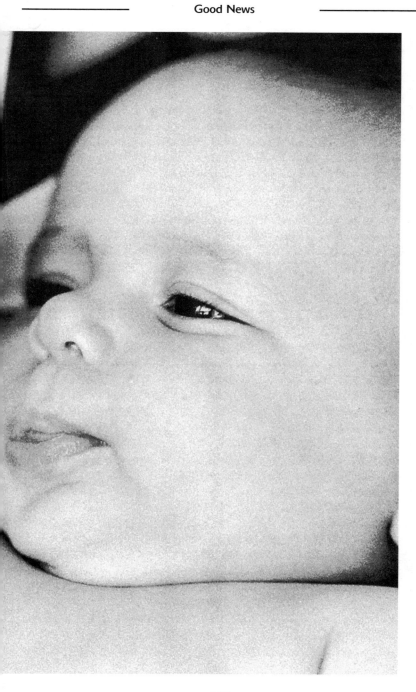

GOOD NEWS

VACCINE UPDATE

Confusion surrounds the vaccination question, and the debate continues. Some illnesses that we routinely vaccinate against are virtually nonexistent in this country. Diphtheria is apparently absent from the US, with no cases reported in 1986. Only three cases had been reported in the two years previous to that. Reported tetanus cases totaled 61 in 1986, and only two cases of paralytic poliomyelitis were reported in 1986.

Pertussis, however, despite near universal vaccination, was more prevalent in 1986 than in any year since 1970. The 1986 total number of pertussis cases was approximately 4,500, with nearly a third of them—1,300 cases—reported in a major outbreak in Kansas. (All 1986 statistics cited above are from the provisional data compiled by the Centers for Disease Control and reported in *Vaccine Bulletin*, February 1987, pp. 11–12.)

This outbreak of pertussis in Kansas occurred in a highly immunized population: "Some 90 percent of the pertussis patients whose immunization status was known, appear to have been adequately immunized." (*Vaccine Bulletin*, February 1987, p. 11) The outbreak affected all age groups—from 0 to 79 years—with most cases concentrated in those under 20 years of age. More cases than would usually be expected occurred in the five to nine age group, and less than would be expected occurred among infants.

Vaccine complications continue to receive national press coverage. Some attention has been given to the development of a different type of vaccination for pertussis, one that is associated with fewer vaccine-related complications. The pertussis vaccine currently in use in this country is a *whole-cell* vaccine, which contains dead pertussis toxin—that remains biologically active after the bacteria that secrete it have been killed—as well as endotoxin, a protein secreted by a virus or bacteria that can, in large enough quantities, affect the brain or produce shock. Developed several years ago in Japan, the *acellular* pertussis vaccine has all of the bacteria and most of the toxins removed or rendered harmless, and is considered more pure and specific. Although the acellular vaccine must undergo testing in this country and physicians will not have legal access to it for two to three years, some physicians who are concerned about side effects from the whole-cell preparation are using test batches of the new vaccine for their own children or are traveling to Japan or Hong Kong to have their children vaccinated. (*The Santa Fe New Mexican*, 5 April 1987)

Two preliminary studies of the acellular vaccine in the US show promising results. Vanderbilt University School of Medicine has thus far conducted studies on 80 children from 18 to 24 months and from four to six years of age. Both age groups showed antibody production comparable to the old vaccine, but far fewer adverse reactions in terms of fever, fretfulness, abnormal gait, and redness, tenderness, and swelling at the vaccination site. (*HealthFacts*, no. 90, November 1986)

Among the non-Communist countries, only the US, Australia, and Iceland have mandatory pertussis vaccination programs. And yet, the pertussis inoculation is the most toxic of all protective vaccines routinely given to children in their first five years of life. Each year, this vaccine is linked to the deaths of at least 44, and possibly as many as 900, otherwise healthy children. It also causes more lasting brain damage than whooping cough would if children were not immunized. Most of the whooping cough in America now occurs in vaccinated children or in those too young to be immunized. (*The Santa Fe New Mexican*, 5 April 1987)

Both Sweden and Japan experienced an increase in cases of whooping cough after discontinuing mass whole-cell vaccination programs. Japan, now using the acellular vaccine and waiting until two years of age to begin vaccination, has witnessed a dramatic decline in both minor and severe reactions to the vaccine and in cases of whooping cough in general. (*The People's Medical Journal*, December 1986)

Many questions remain to be answered regarding the relationship between vaccinations and the decline of an illness in the general population over time; the effect of vaccinations on the immune system; and the safety of administering particular vaccines in a country in which diseases from the conditions vaccinated against are on the decline and in which large numbers of vaccinated people still contract the disease.

Ellen Kleiner
Good News
Summer 1987

MENINGITIS VACCINE UPDATE

In *Mothering*, no. 39 (Spring 1986), we printed a letter from a reader inquiring about the Hib vaccine, licensed in the US in April 1985 to protect against the leading bacterial cause of meningitis. Since then, more research has shed light on the problem and on the vaccine. Two recent studies have concluded that *Hemophilus influenza* type b does not seem to spread from child to child as readily as doctors suspected. (*New England Journal of Medicine*) Earlier studies indicated that the infant brothers or sisters of a child with meningitis are up to 400 times more likely to contract this illness; however, one of the more recent studies showed that only one child out of 587 who had regular contact with an infected toddler went on to develop the illness.

Vaccine failure is also being investigated. Work is under way to determine why it is that some children who receive the preparation go on to develop meningitis. (*New England Journal of Medicine* 315, 18 December 1986)

All we can conclude at this point is that contact with meningitis is less "risky" than was formerly believed; that the other causes of meningitis (such as pneumococcus, meningococcus, some viruses, and other agents) are not inoculated against in the current vaccine; that the Hib vaccine is not effective in the under-two age group, in which 75 percent of all meningitis cases occur; and that the current vaccine will not protect all children who receive it.

Ellen Kleiner

Good News

Summer 1987

VACCINE REFORM IN ALASKA

Vaccination reform legislation is under way in Alaska. Representative Mike Navarre presented HB 277, an act relating to the inoculation of minors, to the Alaska State House on April 17, 1987. The bill has been referred to the Health, Education, and Social Services Committee and will be reviewed when the House of Representatives reconvenes in January 1988.

This bill has four main components. *Parental Choice:* To allow philosophical objection (parental discretion) on administration of vaccinations without threat of exclusion from a school, preschool, or daycare center. *Parent Immunization Information:* To mandate that each parent receive extensive written information on the risks as well as the benefits of each vaccine before vaccination and with vaccine information provided by the Public Health Department at birth. *Adverse Reaction Reports:* To mandate that all healthcare providers report to the Public Health Department all occurrences of serious adverse reactions resulting from inoculations, and that long-term follow-up investigations be included. *Immunization Records:* To ensure that the vaccine manufacturer and lot number be kept on file for at least three years, and that reactions be recorded in a minor's permanent medical record so that no further doses of questionable vaccine are administered to that minor, even if location of adminis-tration varies.

Alaska Dissatisfied Parents Together (AK-DPT) is requesting that all concerned Alaskan parents contact their representatives and ask them to support HB 277. Address letters to Representative _____, AK State Legislature, Pouch V (MS 3100), Juneau, AK 99811. Public support is the key to passage of this much-needed leg-islation.

Readers interested in learning more about these proceedings may contact: Shannon Kohler, President, AK-DPT, Box 1746, Soldotna, AK 99669.

Ellen Kleiner
Good News
Fall 1987

MENINGITIS VACCINE: CONTROVERSIAL FINDINGS

In the Summer 1987 issue of *Mothering*, we printed an update on the vaccine that was approved by the Federal Drug Administra-tion (FDA) in April 1985 to protect against *Hemophilus influenza* type b (Hib), the leading bacterial cause of meningitis. The Centers for Disease Control (CDC) recommended essentially universal vaccina-tion for children at 24 months of age. This past October, the Infectious Disease Committee of the American Academy of Pediatrics (AAP) approved alternative guidelines: under certain circumstances, physicians may choose not to use this vaccine.

The "certain circumstances" are based on recent studies of the vaccine's efficacy and safety in different parts of the country. Five retrospective studies presented at an FDA workshop this past April showed a "surprising number of meningitis cases" among children who had received the vaccine. And Dan Granoff, a pediatrician at Washington University's Children's Hospital in St. Louis, has commented on the vaccine's "unprecedented regionality." In Minnesota, for example, vaccinated children were *more* likely than nonvaccinated children to become infected with Hib; those who became infected were 86 percent more likely than controls to have been vaccinated. (*Science News* 132, 24 October 1987)

Minnesota State epidemiologist Michael Osterholm claims that, rather than protecting children from meningitis, the Hib vaccine increases the risk of illness. He reported that a Minnesota study of children who had received the vaccine since its introduction in 1985 showed they faced a fivefold increase in the risk of infection by the Hib bacteria. ("Meningitis Risk Seen from Use of Vaccine," *St. Paul Pioneer Press Dispatch*, 21 April 1987) According to Granoff, these findings suggest that the vaccine might best be discontinued in this state.

Previous to this, researchers had never seen such regional variation in a vaccine's effectiveness. The original vaccine trials were conducted in Finland, where a 90 percent effectiveness rate was reported. Follow-up effectiveness trials in the US have ranged from 89 percent in some states to the negative correlation found in Minnesota. Some physicians are now questioning the value of transferring data derived from countries with a homogeneous population to the more genetically diverse US.

Also questionable is a particular person's susceptibility to the infection, regardless of his or her vaccination status. Studies among unvaccinated populations show that certain ethnic groups—blacks, American Indians, and Eskimos—are more susceptible to Hib infection than Caucasians. Other studies reveal that some vaccinated individuals seem completely incapable of mounting immune responses against Hib.

Consequently, new approaches to meningitis protection are under way. One development is a *conjugate vaccine*, which, unlike the original preparation that is made from a polysaccharide fragment of the virus, will link this fragment to "immune system stimulants capable of amplifying antibody production." Researchers are hoping that conjugate vaccines will prove effective in children as young as six months of age. However, conjugate vaccines also have potential problems. One is that they have been pretested in Finland and not in this country. Another is that they have a "window of increased susceptibility" to Hib infection during the first seven days after inoculation. Granoff and others claim this is due to the vaccine's action of temporarily "binding up the body's naturally occurring Hib antibodies."

A second new development is *passive vaccination*. The passive vaccine, designed to provide rapid protection against infection, involves the direct injection of Hib-specific immune proteins (immune globulins) taken from the plasma of previously inoculated adults. The disadvantages are: it is expensive; protection is only temporary, requiring repeated doses; and it involves a human blood product and thus carries a small risk of hepatitis or AIDS contamination. (*Science News* 132, 24 October 1987)

As this issue goes to press, new guidelines are being formulated. On February 17, the AAP released a statement recommending that children receive the new conjugate vaccine (PRPD) at 18 months of age in lieu of the "first-generation" polysaccharide (PRP) vaccine at 24 months. The new vaccine, licensed by the FDA this past December, is expected to be safer and more immunologic, and to offer protection to an additional 5 percent of children. The vaccine is not licensed for use in children under 18 months, an age group that encompasses 70 percent of all meningitis cases. (AAP news release, 17 February 1988)
Ellen Kleiner
Good News
Spring 1988

CHILDHOOD VACCINE EXEMPTIONS

Allowable exemptions to mandatory inoculations come in three forms: medical, religious, and philosophical. Medical exemptions, accepted in all 50 states, require a written statement from a licensed physician indicating that the particular vaccination is contraindicated due to a previous adverse reaction, a family history of reactions, a history of convulsions, neurological disorders, severe allergies, prematurity, or recent illness. Licensed naturopathic physicians in Washington State are now allowed to furnish medical exemptions, as are chiropractors in some states.

Religious exemptions are accepted in all states except West Virginia and Mississippi. Philosophical exemptions, based on a parent's personal beliefs, are permitted in 22 states. This option requires a written statement from the parent indicating that he or she has "a moral conviction opposed to vaccination." (Richard Leviton, "Who Calls the Shots?" *East West Journal*, November 1988)

As more parents claim religious exemptions for their children—particularly in states that do not allow philosophical exemptions—the legal system is having to acknowledge a wider range of beliefs. In a recent New York Federal Court lawsuit (*Levy, et al. v. Northport—East Northport Union Free School District, et al.*), US District Court Judge Leonard Wexler ruled that parents can legally claim an exemption from inoculation based on their own "personal religious beliefs" and need not be members of any particular religious group. The earlier statute, requiring membership in a recognized religious organization, was declared unconstitutional—in violation of the First Amendment of the Constitution.

This case has expanded an individual's rights to refuse vaccination in New York. Now, says attorney James Filenbaum, who filed the suit, the courts will have to determine what constitutes "personal religious beliefs." (*Health Science*, November/December 1988, p. 4)

For information on this ruling, contact attorney James Filenbaum, 300 N. Main Street, Suite 108, Spring Valley, NY 10977; 914-425-8804.

Ellen Kleiner
Good News
Spring 1989

VACCINE UPDATES: DPT, MEASLES, CHICKENPOX

Recent developments in vaccine research provide new food for thought. Data from the Centers for Disease Control (CDC) reaffirm that children receiving the DPT shot are at increased risk of having seizures. The analysts note that seizures may be either febrile (fever-induced) or nonfebrile, and that children most at risk are those who have a first-degree relative with a history of convulsions. According to CDC estimates, if family history alone were used to disqualify children from the inoculation, 5 to 7 percent of youngsters in this country would not receive the DPT. (*The Journal of Pediatrics*, October 1989)

As these findings were going to press, a group of multidisciplinary scientists was convening for a three-day international symposium on pertussis—the "P" in DPT. Participants at the September 28, 1989, Workshop on the Neurological Complications of Pertussis and the Pertussis Vaccine concluded that the current whole-cell pertussis vaccine can cause a wide spectrum of permanent brain damage, ranging from learning disabilities to severe retardation to seizure disorders. According to workshop coordinator John Menkes, MD, a University of California at Los Angeles professor of pediatrics and neurology, the neurological complications are in part prompted by the interaction of pertussis toxin and the endotoxin present in *B. pertussis* bacteria. The scientists also concluded that whereas the vaccine may accelerate symptoms in children with an underlying neurologic disorder, *it can also produce symptoms in children with no preexisting abnormality*. Workshop attendants agreed on the importance of replacing the whole-cell vaccine with either a less toxic acellular vaccine or a genetically engineered preparation. (*Vaccine News* 5, no. 1, Spring 1990, pp. 1, 9) A summary of key findings is available for $2.00 from the National Vaccine Information Center, Dissatisfied Parents Together (DPT), 512 W. Maple Avenue, Vienna, VA 22180; 703-983-DPT3.

Four months later, in a federal review of the pertussis vaccine, an Institute of Medicine panel of medical and public health experts maintained that although the vaccine can worsen preexisting problems and bring to light previously unknown problems, there is "no scientific proof that the vaccine causes severe neurological damage or death." Dissenting parents, lawyers, and others argued that public health officials, in their zealous promotion of mass inoculation to wipe out contagious diseases, are deliberately understating the severe side effects of the DPT vaccine. Jeffrey Schwartz—a Washington lawyer whose daughter's 1984 death was attributed to a vaccine-related seizure—pointed out that more than 1,000 reported cases of severe pertussis vaccine reactions are being brushed off by the medical community as "unscientific" and "anecdotal," and that the government, by withholding information about the danger of the vaccine, has been engaged in "a conspiracy of silence and denial." (*The Santa Fe New Mexican*, 11 January 1990, p. A-2)

On the measles front, in response to the nearly 400 percent increase in measles cases between 1988 and 1989, the American Academy of Pediatrics and the CDC are recommending revaccination of all individuals born after 1957. The reasoning is that "virtually everyone born before then was exposed to the highly contagious disease and is now immune to it," and the single shot most children have received since then "has not eradicated the disease." The two-dose recommendation was prompted by a desire to protect the 2 to 10 percent of children who have failed to respond to the first dose. Recommendations for newborns include a first dose of the vaccine at 15 months and a second dose before entering junior high school. Although physicians say that measles is not serious in most cases, they note that it can "lead to life-threatening complications, including pneumonia and brain damage." (*The New York Times*, 30 July 1989, p. A-20)

The National Vaccine Information Center has raised several questions about the new measles protocol. First, considering the number of measles outbreaks in already-vaccinated high school and college populations, could mass vaccinations have caused the measles virus to become more vaccine-resistant? (And if so, could the new mass vaccination program create strains of even greater resistance?) Second, can revaccination be considered an effective option when no national study has been conducted to evaluate whether or not this two-dose option will provide lifelong immunity? And third, can revaccination be considered safe when no study has assessed whether or not the second dose of vaccine will result in adverse reactions? (*Vaccine News*, p. 9)

Another rash of measles concerns appears in Dr. Lisa Lovett's booklet *Immunity: Why Not Keep It?* Lovett presents documentation showing that since the introduction of the measles vaccine, death due to measles has not decreased, the incidence of pneumonia and demonstrable liver abnormalities has increased (from 3 to 20 percent), and children who die from measles are usually malnourished. She also highlights a 1983 study showing that half of all people with measles in the US had been vaccinated against the disease. For a copy of this 74-page booklet, write to Dr. Lovett at 86 Kooyong Road, Armadale, Victoria, 3242, Australia.

On the horizon is pressure to introduce an experimental chickenpox vaccine for mass use. Members of a Federal Drug Administration (FDA) advisory committee are urging the FDA to approve a vaccine developed a decade ago and containing a live but weakened form of the varicella-zoster virus—the first vaccine designed to produce a lifelong "silent infection" in the body. The vaccine's side effects (including shingles), level of effectiveness (study results vary), and duration of effectiveness are all under question. Several decades of use among children could, in the instance of short-term effectiveness, shift the disease to the adult population, where it is much more serious. The advisory board is reportedly requesting FDA approval and widescale safety and effectiveness studies if the vaccine is approved. (*Vaccine News*, p. 90)

In the past eight years alone, the full set of FDA-approved childhood vaccines has increased in scope and in price. In 1982, public health clinics were charging $6.69 to fully vaccinate a child against measles, mumps, rubella, polio, diphtheria, pertussis, and tetanus. Now, with the addition of a second measles dose and at least one Hib vaccine (to protect against meningitis), public health clinics are charging $91.20. ("Immunizations: Protecting Our Children," AAP memorandum, July 1990)

Ellen Kleiner
Good News
Fall 1990

VACCINITIS

An epidemic of vaccines is on the horizon. Some strains are already in existence and are threatening full-blown outbreaks, while others are in various stages of development or awaiting Food and Drug Administration (FDA) approval.

Concerned that preexisting vaccines are failing to reach large segments of the population, the Centers for Disease Control (CDC) has decided to deliver vaccines to poor children through welfare and nutrition offices. Agency officials suggest that the new program, scheduled to get under way later this year, may be based on a contingency plan—that a family's welfare benefits may depend upon the full inoculation of their children. However, Representative Henry A.

Waxman, chairman of the House Subcommittee on Health and Environment, says it would be wrong to withhold benefits or to force women to get their children vaccinated before the government has made vaccines easily accessible. "If parents really refused to get their children immunized [sic], I can see making a penalty for it, but parents are not refusing," he adds. "We have just made it too difficult for them." (*The New York Times*, 17 March 1991, p. 260)

Children are also being targeted to receive the hepatitis B vaccine, to prevent spread of a disease whose victims are almost always adults. The best way to ensure that adults do not get hepatitis B is to vaccinate them when they are children, says the Immunizations Practices Advisory Committee of the Public Health Service (PHS). "This approach to immunize [sic] children to prevent a serious chronic adult disease has never been tried before," explains Dr. Harold Margolis, chief of CDC's hepatitis branch. Still, according to Dr. Carol Phillips of the American Academy of Pediatrics (AAP) committee on infectious diseases, pediatricians are likely to endorse the vaccine. "If you make this vaccine a volitional thing," says St. Louis hepatitis specialist Dr. Robert Perillo, "it's [the control of hepatitis B] not going to happen." (*The New York Times*, 3 March 1991, p. E-7) The AAP, whose long-range goal is universal vaccination, will be releasing final recommendations sometime this summer. (*Pediatric News*, April 1991, p. 1)

While CDC and AAP officials debate a host of vaccine outreach strategies, the PHS advisory commission is scrambling to keep up with an unexpected backlog of vaccine injuries. The National Vaccine Injury Compensation Program is facing a logistical crisis in its effort to cope with the caseload of injuries and deaths occurring before October 1988, when the program went into effect. According to all accounts, the program's budget of $63 million to cover pre-1988 claims will require substantial funding to cover what may amount to as much as $1.5 billion in awards. (*Pediatric News*, January 1991, p. 1) Estimates of the eventual total cost of awards range as high as $3 billion. (*Pediatric News*, April 1991, p. 3) Already the program has tripled its staff to process the more than 3,200 petitions filed. The average award for injury is $1.2 million, while compensation for death is limited by law to $250,000.(*Pediatric News*, January 1991, p. 35)

Still in the embryonic stages of development are a universal childhood vaccine and a vaccine to prevent pregnancy. Further along and up for FDA approval is an experimental chickenpox vaccine containing a live but weakened form of the varicella zoster virus. This vaccine is said to stimulate a lifelong "silent infection" in the body. Proponents are pushing for a mass vaccination requirement; however, critics argue that the vaccine has been insufficiently tested for safety and effectiveness, and that decades of use in childhood could propel the disease into the adult population, where its consequences would be much more serious. (*Mothering*, no. 57, Fall 1990, p. 87)

Do vaccines make for healthy children? Do more vaccines make for healthier children? How can a parent exercise freedom of choice amid the burgeoning vaccine requirements being proposed by federal panels? Informed-choice advocates say it is time to let federal and state legislators know that enough is enough. When lots of people speak up—via letters to the editors of papers, visits to state representatives, and open dialogues in community forums—lawmakers pay attention.

Good News
Summer 1991

ADVERSE REACTIONS TO THE VACCINE PUSH

Now that physicians in the US are required by the Childhood Vaccine Injury Act of 1986 to report adverse reactions to childhood inoculations, official numbers are pouring in. According to the FDA register, between November 1990 and August 1992 more than 300 children died and more than 17,000 were adversely affected as a direct result of one of the five commonly administered vaccines: the DPT (diphtheria, pertussis, tetanus) vaccine, the MMR (measles, mumps, rubella) vaccine, the oral polio vaccine, the hepatitis B vaccine, and the Hemophilus B conjugate (Hib) vaccine against viral meningitis. "Adverse reactions" are defined as shock, seizures and convulsions, brain damage, or any condition of illness, disability, or injury arising within approximately 72 hours of inoculation.

Evidence linking adverse reactions to the vaccines themselves is insufficient to warrant any change in recommendation, says Michael Copeland, spokesperson for the American Academy of Pediatrics (AAP). Holding to this perception, the AAP continues to advise routine vaccination against these five diseases, only four of which are related to childhood. Increasing numbers of pediatricians are jumping on the bandwagon, and states are expanding their mandates to encompass the growing number of "advisable" vaccines.

Critics, meanwhile, are exhibiting adverse reactions of their own. Joanne M. Hatem, MD, medical director of the consumer-based National Vaccine Information Center, argues that not all doctors are complying with reporting regulations, and that FDA statistics represent only about 10 percent of adverse reactions to the vaccines. (*Vegetarian Times*, February 1993, p. 16) Terence J. Bovill, of the Health Research Foundation in Gloucestershire, England, warns that vaccines endanger lives by introducing foreign proteins that the body can process only at great expense to vital organs. He maintains that although "there is not a shred of evidence that [vaccination] either prevents or reduces the effects of any disease for which it is intended . . . [it remains] acceptable to both governments and doctors alike because of the high financial rewards involved." (*Health Consciousness* 13, no. 5, 1992, p. 58) Parents, who are no happier with recent developments, are objecting to compulsory inoculations for a variety of reasons, including individual health concerns, religious or personal beliefs, prior experience with particular serums, and familiarity with postvaccination episodes in the lives of children they know or knew.

To assist parents in search of legal options to compulsory inoculations, New York attorney and longtime health-freedom advocate James R. Filenbaum has established a toll-free hotline: 1-800-753-5297. For material on the physiological effects of the various vaccines, or to receive a DPT information packet, contact the National Vaccine Information Center, at 512 W. Maple Avenue #206, Vienna, VA 22180; or call 703-938-3783. To share your views and experiences with the nation's committee on healthcare reform, write to Hillary Rodham Clinton, 1600 Pennsylvania Avenue NW, Washington, DC 20500.

Good News
Fall 1993

VACCINE UPDATE

On July 31, 1996, the Food and Drug Administration (FDA) licensed an acellular pertussis vaccine for babies under 18 months old. The acellular pertussis vaccine is less reactive than the whole-cell pertussis vaccine. Vaccine activists have called for the total removal of the whole-cell pertussis vaccine.

Japan has been using an acellular vaccine begun at age two to control whooping cough since 1981. At a June 20, 1996, meeting of the Advisory Committee on Immunization Practices (ACIP) of the Centers for Disease Control (CDC), members of the federal vaccine policy-making panel voted to move away from use of the live oral polio vaccine (OPV). Instead, they opted for the increased use of the injectable inactivated polio vaccine (IPV), in order to decrease the number of polio cases caused by OPV.

The US has been vaccinating with oral polio for 32 years. Wild polio disease has been eliminated from the Western Hemisphere by OPV, which is now the only cause of polio in the country today. Be cautious about coming in contact with the bodily fluids of a person who has recently swallowed live OPV.

The workshop summary of the Vaccine Safety Forum, *Options for Poliomyelitis Vaccination in the United States*, is available from the Institute of Medicine, National Academy Press, 2101 Constitution Avenue NW, Washington, DC 20418. 202-334-3935.

Good News
Winter 1996

CHILDHOOD DISEASES

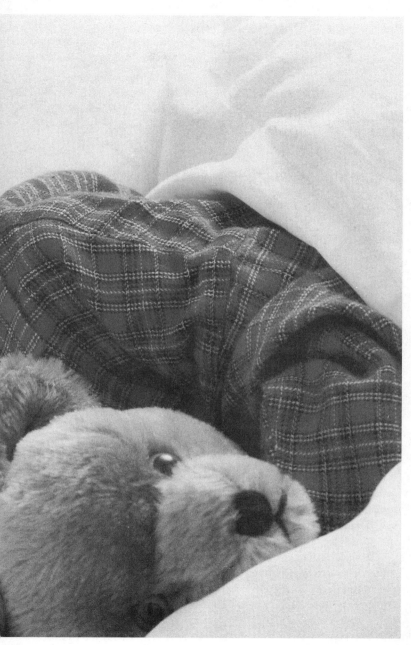

WHOOPING COUGH
BY ANNA JOYCE

Anna Joyce is a marriage and family therapist currently staying home as a full-time mom. She lives with her husband, Marty, a psychiatrist, and their three children: Erika, Daniel, and Matt, who was born happy and healthy, with no complications. The family lives in Benicia, California.

I was seven months pregnant with our third child when my husband started coughing. Since it was allergy season in northern California, we didn't pay much attention. Marty described it as a "tickle sensation" in the back of his throat, accompanied by a runny nose and postnasal drip that triggered the dry, tight cough. A week later, when the cough had not subsided and he was feeling more depleted, he visited a family practitioner. The diagnosis was either an allergy or a viral cough, something that had been "going around" lately. Several days later, however, the cough suddenly turned into a long, paroxysmal, racking cough punctuated by wheezy "whooping" sounds as Marty struggled for air. We rechecked with our family doctor, who said that his type of "whooping" can be present in viral illnesses, but considered asthma as another possibility. He sent Marty to the outpatient clinic of our local hospital for blood tests and broncho-dilation, but the tests were negative and showed no elevated white cell count such as might be found in a bacterial infection. Virus, they all said.

I was in a mild state of panic. We had an unvaccinated two year old, and I thought that Marty's cough seemed unnervingly similar to descriptions I had read of whooping cough. I asked our doctor to order a pertussis culture at the public health department. Despite all indications to the contrary, he agreed and four days later called to say, "I can't believe it, but the public health department just called me—Marty's culture *is* growing out pertussis."

A wave of fear and sadness swept over me as I hung up the phone. Our two year old had been coughing for about five days, a mild nondescript cough of the sort commonly heard in schoolrooms and grocery stores. But it was too coincidental. I feared he was developing whooping cough, too.

The day that I requested the culture on my husband, I also

called our pediatrician to request a prescription for prophylactic antibiotics for our son Daniel (erythromycin being the drug of choice for pertussis). Our pediatrician resisted my suggestion, as he was critical of my earlier choice not to vaccinate Daniel, and I learned an important lesson: working with a health practitioner who is not comfortable with parents' rights to make informed, independent choices that sometimes go against his or her advice is risky business. This marked the end of our relationship with our pediatrician, and we later learned that immediately treating Daniel with erythromycin would have been the wisest course of action. In the future, I will remember the power of a mother's intuition.

After the initial shock of the culture results wore off, we mobilized ourselves and began gathering information about pertussis. Given its rarity during the past decade or two, this was not an easy task. We consulted with the following sources, who offered frequent contradictions: a family practitioner; an old-time pediatrician who had seen many cases of pertussis; a young pediatrician with a specialty in infectious diseases; an infectious disease specialist who currently treated only adults; a pediatrician in the infectious disease department of Childrens' Hospital in Oakland, California; a pediatrician specializing in infectious diseases at Stanford Medical Center in Palo Alto, California; a pediatrician from the Kaiser System, who in turn contacted a UCLA research physician considered to be the West Coast authority on pertussis; and a public health official from Solano County, California, who visited our home.

Pertussis runs its course in about six weeks. The first two weeks are the *prodrome*, during which time the symptoms are a runny nose, congestion, and a rather ordinary cough. A diagnosis at this stage is nearly impossible without a culture, and culturing often appears unnecessary. In addition, the cultures are difficult to read, and culturing too early can produce false-negative results. The third and fourth weeks are the severe stage of the illness. During this time, the characteristic "whoop" emerges, along with paroxysmal coughing that can be accompanied by vomiting, cyanosis (bluish discoloration of skin and mucous membranes), and in the worst cases: brain hemorrhage, broken ribs, or damaged lungs from the force of coughing. My husband, Marty, had pulled muscles and bruised ribs from coughing so hard. The final two weeks are the convalescent stage of the illness, during which time the severe symptoms abate in frequency and intensity.

The nature of the disease process makes treatment of pertussis difficult. While the bacteria, *Bordetella pertussis* is actually very responsive to erythromycin, the bacteria produces an endotoxin that is not responsive. The erythromycin will usually eradicate the bacteria within the first five days of treatment (although a 14-day course of treatment is considered essential to avoid relapse), but the medication does not affect the damage done by the toxin. The toxin irritates and congests the respiratory system, and triggers the cough center in the brain. The person with pertussis continues to experience the same level of symptomatology after several days of antibiotic treatment. The disease may progress no further once the bacteria is killed, but will continue to run its four- to six-week course.

Early intervention with erythromycin, however, can abort or minimize the course of the illness. In Daniel's case, because we began treatment before he reached the paroxysmal stage, the illness was fairly mild. He never experienced the severe spasms of coughing, gasping for air, and turning blue that characterize the more serious cases. The public health nurse, the infectious disease specialist, and the pediatrician at Childrens' Hospital all predicted accurately that his symptoms would level off after approximately five days of antibiotic treatment.

In my case, we were especially concerned because of my pregnancy. The night that I began the antibiotics, I awoke with a sore throat, and by the next morning I had a full-blown cold. By the following day, I had developed a tight cough that was very painful and pulled on my abdominal muscles. My symptoms progressed no further.

We supplemented the antibiotic treatment with naturopathic and homeopathic care under the direction of specialists in these fields. We took echinacea and goldenseal; large doses of vitamins C and A; zinc supplements; flower pollen supplements; and lactobacillus to counteract the effects of the erythromycin on the digestive tract.

The homeopathic remedies we used were the cell salt *Magnesia phosphorica*, *Drosera* for my husband and son, *Pulsatilla* for me, and *Spongia* for my nine-year-old daughter. We all took *Pertussin* 30c once daily.

Looking back, I would not forgo *any* of the three courses of treatment we chose. We take antibiotics infrequently, only after other options have been unsuccessful, but I will always be grateful for the availability of an antibiotic that helped to minimize the course of illness for all of us.

While I do not regret our decision not to vaccinate our son Daniel, I have a greater appreciation for the fear of pertussis that many health practitioners hold. I am certain that watching a child experience a severe case of whooping cough is very painful.

We now await the birth of our newborn. Some medical practitioners advise that we should all be recultured before the birth, and that if any of us culture positively, that person should be retreated with antibiotics and the baby should be treated as well. If we all culture negatively, the UCLA specialist recommends watching the baby closely for signs of respiratory infection during the first few months, and giving erythromycin "just in case."

I believe that taking the responsibility for the health care of yourself and your family is a big responsibility. If you choose not to vaccinate, it is imperative to learn as much as possible about the disease you are not vaccinating against as well as other life-threatening diseases. I also believe that it is important to choose health professionals with whom you are philosophically compatible and who are willing to help in times of crisis.

HELPFUL INFORMATION
BY ANNA JOYCE

Early intervention with erythromycin *can* impact the course of pertussis. If you know your child has been exposed, he or she can be given this antibiotic prophylactically. My in-laws, who had total exposure to us because they spent a lot of time at our house cleaning, cooking, and helping during the crisis, took the medication and did not contract pertussis. Another family, who had been with us prior to diagnosis, developed mild, coldlike symptoms, but they, too, took the medication and their symptoms did not progress further.

The culture for pertussis is best taken through the nose and sinus passages. The old method of having the person cough onto a culture plate resulted in many false negatives.

Some forms of erythromycin are more effective than others. The *estolate* is considered most reliable, providing the least incidence of relapse or positive culture following treatment. *Ilosone*, the liquid form of erythromycin given to children, is an estolate. The succinate variety is generally considered least effective.

My nine-year-old daughter had been fully vaccinated, but consensus in the medical community is that immunity lasts for only three to five years. One pediatrician we contacted had recently treated fully immunized young children who had contracted pertussis. Other reports also question the effectiveness of the vaccine. However, my daughter developed only a mild case of the illness.

Most health practitioners agree that it is primarily children under one year of age who are at greatest risk from pertussis and who are most likely to be hospitalized or suffer complications.

Homeopathy has had great success in treating pertussis with the nosode *Pertussin*. However, since we chose antibiotic treatment as well, I am unable to personally say how effective homeopathy would be alone. The homeopathic remedies we took did alleviate the symptoms after the antibiotic destroyed the bacteria.

NATURAL REMEDIES FOR CHILDHOOD DISEASES
BY MIRANDA CASTRO

Miranda Castro, FS Hom, CCH, is the author of The Complete Homeopathy Handbook *and* Homeopathy for Pregnancy, Birth, and Your Baby's First Year, *both from St. Martin's Press. Her son was raised exclusively on homeopathy and TLC. "Natural Remedies for Childhood Diseases" first appeared in* Mothering, *no. 77 (Winter 1995).*

Your child has just been diagnosed as having chickenpox or even German measles or mumps (they *are* still around in spite of vaccinations), and your doctor has prescribed Tylenol (acetaminophen) for the fever. This may be your child's first "real" illness apart from the odd minor cough or cold, and you don't know how you are going to cope. Illness can be scary, especially for new parents. There is a fear of not being in control, of something serious happening to your child's health, and of it costing time or money— or both. These fears are made more acute by your child's vulnerability and young age.

Don't panic! Homeopaths believe that these illnesses are not all bad. We see them as an opportunity for the immune system to develop strength and resistance, especially to inherited weaknesses. Children who have come through a childhood illness successfully are seen to be stronger afterwards and often have a growth spurt— either physically and/or mentally and emotionally. My son, Daniel, grew a whole inch in the month after he had measles, and teachers remarked on how much better he was doing in school!

I remember a patient—I'll call her Susan—who telephoned me late one evening in a terrible state. Her one-year-old son, David, had chickenpox. He also had a runny nose, a cough, and a fever—his first illness and first fever. Susan was awash with fear and panic. She hadn't wanted to bother me, as David had seemed to be coping quite well for a while, but in the last few hours his fever had risen to 101°F, and he hadn't eaten his dinner. What Susan needed was some basic information about childhood illnesses and reassurance. I explained that 101°F was a fairly low-grade fever, and it was perfectly normal for a fever to rise in the evening. I added that it was fine he wasn't hungry.

She was desperate to give her baby something to make him well—Tylenol for the fever, cough medicine, painkillers, or at least a homeopathic medicine. But despite the fever, David was basically dealing with his illness well; he was sleeping a lot more than usual (Susan was relieved to hear that this was both normal and healthy), he was drinking plenty, and producing a lot of wet diapers. I asked Susan whether she could take time off from work. She could. I then asked how she and her husband felt about having their son sleep with them. I told her that the thing her child needed most was tender, loving care. She and her husband could tuck David into bed with them, since children often sleep better snuggled up to a parent when they are ill. I suggested that we wait till the morning before prescribing to see what his body could do to heal itself. I warned her that his fever could rise even more and told her not to worry as long as it stayed under 104°F. She should offer water every time he woke and take his clothes off only if he felt hot and sweaty. Susan was relieved but cautious. I told her to talk to David, to reassure him about what was happening, and to validate his ability to heal himself.

In the morning Susan called with joy in her voice. They had all had a rough night; David's fever had gone up to 103°F around midnight, and he had slept restlessly. But after about 2:00 a.m. he had slept for an uninterrupted four hours and had awakened with a big smile on his face and no fever, asking for breakfast. Apart from a little cough, he was just fine.

Susan felt so proud of herself and her son. It was enormously empowering for her to have been so instrumental in her son's healing and to witness his ability to heal himself. I suggested they take it easy and have some fun at home, and not to worry if the fever rose again in the evening. This mother now has a skill for life for dealing with illness in her family.

It is important to put this story into perspective. There are times when our children's illnesses do require urgent medical attention. I believe that parents "know" instinctively when something is seriously wrong with their children and when they need urgent medical help. There have been times in my practice when I have responded to a call from a parent whose child's illness was more serious than little David's. At the same time I believe that it's important for healthcare professionals like myself to know both when to step in and when to step back. While I don't want to lull parents into a false sense of security, I do want to redress the balance somewhat away from the current panic approach.

LOOKING AFTER YOURSELF

If you are a working parent, you will need to prepare yourself for the fact that your children will fall ill from time to time, especially after they start daycare or school. Inevitably, they will need looking after, either by you or by someone else who cares. It's worthwhile to plan ahead for the possibility of illness and to develop strategies for coping. If you aren't prepared, it is easy to feel harassed and resentful when a child does fall ill. And the more children you have, the more prepared you will need to be, since they can fall ill one after the other instead of conveniently all at once!

Engage the help of neighbors, friends, or family to look after your child so that you can rest or get out to recharge your own batteries. Negotiate carefully with your partner so that both of you can get some time off. Take turns doing night duty or split the night into two so that you can both get a good chunk of sleep. Looking after a sick child is draining, especially if your child is very ill or demanding. Now is not the time to worry about whether your house is neat and tidy; ditch the housework for the moment and spend your time off doing something enjoyable or restful, or both! Take a walk, meet with a friend, have a long, hot, uninterrupted bath. Make sure your own cup is full(ish) so that you can give to your child and still have some left over for yourself.

There is a modern myth that tells us illness is a bad thing. The pressure people put on themselves to be well all of the time, often because they cannot afford to take time off, is stress-inducing and needs questioning. This pressure can be projected onto our children—a pressure for parents to get it right, to do a perfect job, to have children who are always well and happy. I believe this is unrealistic and untenable. Many parents and children take medication in order to get back to work—or school—as fast as they possibly can, but this can create a different set of long-term health problems, which can take significantly longer to deal with. When our children are sick, this desire to be a perfect parent tends to get in the way, since children cannot be reasonably well and happy all of the time.

The bottom line is that illness is part of life's rich tapestry, and that includes childhood illnesses. Tampering with nature is not always successful—older children and young adults who contract illnesses "meant" for younger children tend to get more severe attacks. Young men who get mumps have an added risk of infertility because the testes can be affected. Further, it's not entirely unreasonable to expose your child to a friend who has a childhood illness, as *there is no real substitute for natural immunity*.

NURSING A SICK CHILD

It's becoming increasingly common to give sick children Tylenol and then encourage them to carry on a normal life. This is wrong. Our bodies need to slow down and rest as much as possible to encourage our immune system to get to work. It isn't an old wives' tale that the healing activities of the body—the repair, renewal, and growth of cells—actually speed up when we sleep.

Think back to your own childhood. How did your parents care for you when you were sick? Was it a pleasure? A time when everything slowed down, a time of extra cuddles, stories in bed, and special, soothing drinks? If so, you have a rich store of memories to draw upon to help you with your children when they are ill. If you were unlucky, if illness was an inconvenience, or if you were dealt with harshly when you were ill, then you may want to think carefully so as not to inadvertently repeat your parents' mistakes. The art of nursing a sick child through an illness needs resurrecting. Sick children deserve special treatment—reassurance if they are frightened; comforting if they are in pain; distracting if they have an itchy rash; sponging down if they are too hot. Many parents love this nurturing time when their children are willing and eager to "lean into them."

Encourage bed rest for a sick child. Make up a bed on the sitting room sofa in the daytime so that your child doesn't feel shut off from family life. Keep excitement levels down and encourage quiet activities such as reading, drawing, playing board games, watching a little television (too much is overstimulating), and listening to music and stories. Don't overstimulate sick children by taking them out or by having a lot of visitors.

Make sure your child gets lots of extra sleep (with early nights and daytime naps). If necessary, lie down with your child while he or she sleeps, and let your child sleep with you at night if he or she wants to. Some babies when sick will only sleep well if their mother's body is close to theirs. Use this time to catch up on some sleep or reading.

Small children who develop fevers, especially infants under six months old, must be watched carefully because they are likely to become quickly dehydrated. Encourage all sick children to drink plenty of fluids, preferably water, herb teas, or diluted fruit juice (not sweet or fizzy drinks, as sugar is a stimulant), either warm or cold as desired. Don't give acidic drinks (orange or lemon juice) to a child with mumps, as they will irritate sore salivary glands. Children who are reluctant to drink will often suck on a wet sponge or washcloth, especially if the water is warm, or try an ice cube or frozen fruit juice. If you are breastfeeding a sick baby, continue to nurse as often as your baby asks. The breast is comforting at a time like this.

Don't encourage sick children to eat, especially if they don't want to. Fasting encourages the body in its process of healing. Give hungry children small, light, nutritious meals such as fruit or vegetable purées, soups, and porridge.

Finally, talk reassuringly to your children about what is happening. The sound of your voice will be comforting to them. Explain clearly (even to a baby) what is wrong, and let them know how long the illness is likely to go on. Children who are sick can become more demanding and regress temporarily, sucking things, wetting the bed, and so on—sometimes even before the symptoms of the illness (e.g., rashes, swollen glands) appear. Be patient with them; this will pass once they are on the road to recovery.

DEALING WITH THE FEVER

A fever is often the first symptom to let you know that your child is ill. It's a helpful and necessary part of the process of healing in a childhood illness, since during a fever the healing reactions of the body are speeded up; the heart beats faster, carrying the blood more quickly to all the organs; respiration is quicker, increasing oxygen intake; and perspiration increases, helping the body to cool down naturally. A high temperature generally indicates that the body's defense mechanism is fighting an infection, and temperature variations indicate how it is coping. Attempts to suppress or control a fever artificially with Tylenol, or even with homeopathic remedies, are likely to confuse the body's natural efforts to heal itself. It is best to wait for other symptoms to develop before giving a homeopathic remedy.

Each person has her or his own pattern of falling ill and will experience different fever symptoms. Some people may feel hot with a high fever, but their skin will feel chilly. Others may be irritable, intolerant of any disturbance, and need to be kept warm, while still others may be aching and restless. One person may sweat profusely, be thirsty and slightly delirious; another may want company, while another will prefer to be alone. Each person with a fever may need a different homeopathic remedy, depending on her or his emotional state and general symptoms.

The average normal temperature in a healthy human is said to be 98.6°F (37°C), but this can vary quite markedly. Most people, adults and children, can run a fever of up to 104°F (40°C) for several days with no danger. It is normal for an infection to cause otherwise healthy infants and children to run high fevers of 103°F (39.5°C) and over. A temperature of 105°F (40.5°C) is a serious cause for concern, but only when it surpasses 106°F (41°C) is there a risk to life.

Fevers usually peak toward nighttime and drop by the following morning, so a temperature of 104°F (40°C) registered in the evening may recur on subsequent evenings. A drop in temperature in the morning does not mean that the fever is past its peak. It can rise and fall several times over several days before finally returning to normal. Although a child whose temperature soars may look and feel very ill, therefore giving more cause for concern, such a child is usually ill for a shorter time and recovers sooner than one whose temperature is lower. My friend Maggi's youngest boy always falls ill in a sudden and dramatic fashion. With the mumps, his temperature soared to over 105°F, and he was in a lot of pain from swollen glands. Homeopathy alleviated the pain; he slept and drank a lot and was over his mumps in two days with no further homeopathic assistance. With one of his sisters, it took several days for the mumps to appear, and her temperature never rose above 101°F. She was ill for a week altogether and needed *Pulsatilla* and *Phosphorus* to help her recover.

If the fever goes above 103° to 104°F (40°C) and the skin feels hot and sweaty, sponge your child down with tepid water. Expose and sponge one limb at a time until it feels cool to the touch. Dry and replace it under the covers before going on to the next limb. This will help the temperature to drop by 1 to 2°F (up to 1°C) and can be repeated as often as necessary. Sponging the face and fore-head alone can also give relief. Or you can immerse a feverish but not desperately ill child in a bath from time to time to bring down a high fever. In any case, keep a hot, feverish child cool, and a chilly, feverish child (one who feels cold to the touch and shivers) warm.

Never give a child aspirin in any form during or after a childhood illness, as this can cause serious complications. Use Tylenol in an emergency, when the temperature rises above 104°F (40°C) and sponging hasn't worked, or if your child is in pain and you don't have a homeopathic remedy immediately on hand.

CONVALESCENCE

Once the acute symptoms are over, it's important to take things easy until your child has fully recovered his or her strength and vitality, especially after one of the more serious childhood illnesses such as whooping cough or measles. It is not uncommon for complications, such as a cough or earache, to develop just when you thought everything was back to normal. Keep your child at home until she or he is eating and sleeping normally.

HOW CAN HOMEOPATHY HELP?

Homeopathic treatment will help at all stages of a childhood illness, particularly in addressing an itchy rash or painful swollen glands, an accompanying cough, or sore, dry eyes. Antibiotic treatment is useless for viral infections (except scarlet fever) and will only add to your child's stress load. Avoid it during this time and use homeopathic medicines to stimulate your child's immune system.

SEEK HELP IF:

• your feverish, sick child (especially a baby under six months old) has become lethargic and is drinking less than usual or refusing drinks.

• a baby under six months old has a fever.

• an older baby has a fever of over 104° F (40° C) that doesn't respond to sponging and/or homeopathic treatment within 24 hours.

• there is a lack of reaction (listlessness and limpness), which can imply that a serious illness such as pneumonia or meningitis has developed.

• your child is screaming and is obviously in pain, but you don't know where.

• a rash becomes infected.

A child who doesn't recover well from a childhood illness should seek constitutional treatment from a homeopathic practitioner.

CHILDHOOD DISEASES AT A GLANCE

CHICKENPOX
Incubation: 7–21 days
Infectious Period: A few days before the rash until the last spot or blister has formed a scab
Chickenpox starts with a fever, loss of appetite, and some irritability. As the spots come out, they form itchy blisters that go through a pustular stage before crusting over. Dress your child in loose cotton clothes and cut his or her fingernails (use mitts on a baby) to prevent scratching, especially as chickenpox rash can leave scars.

MUMPS
Incubation: 12–28 days
Infectious Period: 2 days before swelling of glands appears until swelling subsides
Mumps usually occurs as a mild childhood infection, especially in infants. The most common (and often the first) symptom is the swelling of one or both of the salivary glands (in front of the ear and just above the angle of the jaw). The glands under the tongue and jaw may also swell. Give drinks through a straw or from a bottle if it is painful to open the mouth. Wrap a hot water bottle in a towel and let your child lie on it to soothe painful swellings.

GERMAN MEASLES (RUBELLA)
Incubation: 14–21 days
Infectious Period: 5 days before and 7 days after rash appears
German measles, or rubella, is generally a short-lived, mild infection. A faint pink rash of tiny spots starts behind the ears or on the face and spreads down the body. It may be accompanied by

watery eyes and swollen glands at the back of the neck and/or behind the ears, under the arms, or in the groin. Fever rarely goes above 101°F. Do avoid contact with pregnant women while your child has German measles and notify pregnant women with whom or with whose children you were in contact in the three-week period before the spots came out.

MEASLES

Incubation: 8–21 days

Infectious Period: 4 days before and 5–10 days after rash

If you suspect your baby is incubating measles, look for small spots like grains of sand (known as Koplick's spots) in the mouth and inside the cheeks. Measles lasts up to two weeks. It starts with a high fever and watery, red eyes that are sensitive to light. The rash—blotchy and itchy with raised spots—will appear a few days later, starting behind the ears and spreading down the body. As it spreads, the fever will begin to drop. Keep a child with measles and sore eyes out of bright light, with curtains partially closed and lights dimmed.

ROSEOLA

Incubation: 5–15 days

Infectious Period: unknown

Roseola is a mild infectious illness that rarely needs treating. The rash is very similar to German measles, and the two are sometimes confused. In German measles the rash appears with the fever, and in roseola it appears when the fever has come down.

SCARLET FEVER

Incubation: 7–21 days

Infectious Period: 7 days after rash appears

This highly infectious disease is caused by the *Streptococcus* bacteria. The symptoms are a sore throat, followed a day or two later by a rash of tiny spots, beginning on the neck and chest and spreading over the whole body, giving the skin a texture like sandpaper. Other symptoms include vomiting, fever, and a flushed face (though the area around the mouth may be pale). The tongue may also have a red and white "strawberry" appearance. It is important that you consult your doctor if you suspect your child has scarlet fever.

WHOOPING COUGH

Incubation: 7–21 days

Infectious Period: Up to 3–4 weeks after the illness appears

The first signs of whooping cough are a slight fever and runny nose. These are followed by a loose cough. The mucus then thickens, resulting in extended, uncontrollable coughing fits, after which the child draws air convulsively back into the lungs, causing the characteristic "whoop." Whooping cough is often accompanied by retching and/or vomiting.

Young babies may not be able to inhale properly after a coughing fit and may also find eating difficult if they vomit frequently. Get professional help if home prescribing does not produce a quick response.

Whooping cough can last from three weeks to all winter long and is a long and exhausting infection for both child and parent.

HOMEOPATHY AND CHILDHOOD ILLNESSES

Consider the following as a basic guide to home prescribing for childhood diseases. For a fuller description of these remedies, you may want to consult a homeopathic first-aid book. If your child's symptoms don't fit one of the portraits below, you can always seek the advice of a professional homeopath.

Symptoms: Restless, anxious, chilly children who want to be covered. They are terribly weak and only want hot drinks, which they will drink a sip at a time.

Remedy: *Arsenicum*

Diseases: Measles, Mumps, Scarlet Fever

Symptoms: Illness starts suddenly and is accompanied by a high fever, runny nose, dry, croupy cough, reddened, sore eyes, and/or a sore throat. Rashes burn and itch. Children are restless, anxious, and afraid, especially of dying. They are generally thirsty for cold water, don't like warmth, and at night prefer to be uncovered.

Remedy: *Aconite*

Diseases: Chickenpox, German Measles, Measles, Scarlet Fever, Whooping Cough

Symptoms: The rash is slow to come out, and when it does it itches and stings. Affected parts (e.g., rash, glands) are puffy and also itch and sting. Children are extremely restless, anxious, and clingy. They are generally thirstless, don't like to be touched, and prefer cool air and cool bathing to heat.
Remedy: *Apis*
Diseases: Measles, Mumps, Scarlet Fever

Symptoms: Chickenpox, during which the rash is slow to come out. Children are irritable and drowsy. They are sweaty and nauseous and develop a stubborn cough that's loose and rattling. There is a lot of mucus that can't be brought up.
Remedy: *Antimonium tartaricum*
Diseases: Chickenpox, Whooping Cough

Symptoms: Illness is accompanied by a tickling cough and nausea. Children are sulky and extremely irritable; they do not want to be touched or examined, or even looked at. The tongue is white, as if it has been painted.
Remedy: *Antimonium crudum*
Disease: Measles

Symptoms: Whooping cough with a choking, racking, tickling cough. Coughing fits end in retching and coughing up mucus, which hangs in strings. Children generally don't like stuffy rooms and around midnight feel better in fresh air.
Remedy: *Coccus cacti*
Disease: Whooping Cough

Symptoms: The illness starts suddenly and can be accompanied by bed-wetting, a runny nose, cough, sore throat, a throbbing headache, and/or burning, dry, red eyes. The pupils are dilated, and the tongue is red with white spots (like a strawberry). The rash is red, hot, dry, and very itchy. Children are restless, irritable, and sometimes delirious with a high fever. They are generally thirstless, disliking noise and touch, appreciating rest and warmth.
Remedy: *Belladonna*
Diseases: Chickenpox, German Measles, Measles, Mumps, Scarlet Fever, Whooping Cough

Symptoms: Any childhood illness where the rash is slow to appear or doesn't come out fully. There may also be a dry, painful cough that is made worse by movement. Children are irritable and want to be left alone. They are generally thirsty for large quantities of liquid (and gulp them) at infrequent intervals.
Remedy: *Bryonia*
Diseases: German Measles, Measles, Mumps, Scarlet Fever, Whooping Cough

Symptoms: Whooping cough (or cough after measles) with severe, violent cough as well as vomiting and nosebleeds. Face may go blue with each coughing fit. Voice becomes hoarse. The cough is worse when lying down, talking, or laughing; better with fresh air.
Remedy: *Drosera*
Disease: Whooping Cough

Symptoms: Measles where the rash is slow to come out and there is a constant nausea (with a clear, red tongue) that isn't relieved by vomiting. There is a dry cough that comes in fits and ends in choking and gagging. Children are hard to please, generally thirstless; made worse by heat.
Remedy: *Ipecacuanha*
Disease: Measles

Symptoms: Measles with very sore, swollen, sensitive, watery eyes. Nose streams but does not irritate. There may be a harsh cough and headache.
Remedy: *Euphrasia*
Disease: Measles

Symptoms: Measles that come on slowly in warm weather with cold or flulike symptoms accompanied by a great weariness and heaviness. The eyes are swollen and watery. Children are generally apathetic, thirstless, and feverish with chills.
Remedy: *Gelsemium*
Disease: Measles

Symptoms: Mumps with exhaustion. Glands swollen, making swallowing and talking difficult. Profuse sweating and salivation.

Breasts, ovaries, or testicles become painful. Generally thirsty; made worse by cold.

Remedy: *Jaborandi*

Disease: Mumps

Symptoms: Swollen, painful glands. Pains shoot to ears and/or neck. Illness may be accompanied by a runny nose, earache, sticky eyes, and sore throat. Profuse, smelly sweating, and salivation. Metallic taste in mouth (may have mouth ulcers) and smelly breath. Generally feels worse at night, with extremes of temperature and sweating; feels better with rest.

Remedy: *Mercurius*

Diseases: Chickenpox, German Measles, Measles, Mumps, Scarlet Fever

Symptoms: For the later stages of measles where there is stubborn inflammation of mucus membranes, with swollen glands and deafness from inflammation in the eustachian tubes.

Remedy: *Kali bichromicum*

Disease: Measles

Symptoms: The illness is accompanied by swollen glands, thick, yellow mucus, bedwetting, a dry cough at night and loose cough in the morning, sticky eyes, earache, and/or a fever. In mumps the breasts, ovaries, or testicles are painful. Children are weepy, whiny, and clingy. Small children want to be carried everywhere. They are generally thirstless; feel worse in heat and when lying down at night; better in fresh air.

Remedy: *Pulsatilla*

Diseases: Chickenpox, German Measles, Measles, Mumps, Whooping Cough

Symptoms: Illness is accompanied by swollen glands, aching joints, and/or sore eyes. The rash is very itchy and causes great restlessness. The tongue has a red tip. Children are depressed. They are generally worse with cold and at night; better with warmth, particularly with a hot bath.

Remedy: *Rhus tox*

Diseases: Chickenpox, German Measles, Measles, Mumps, Scarlet Fever

Symptoms: Illness is accompanied by bedwetting, earache (left side), sore, red eyes, fever, and/or runny nose. Tongue is white with a red tip and edges. Rash is red, hot, and itches maddeningly. Children are restless and irritable. They are generally thirsty for cold drinks (usually water); uncomfortable with heat and bathing; better with fresh air.

Remedy: *Sulphur*

Diseases: Chickenpox, German Measles, Measles, Scarlet Fever

This is a rough guide. If your child has, for example, mumps and is exhibiting strong guiding symptoms for *Pulsatilla*, you can give it even though it isn't a big mumps remedy. The important thing is to treat the whole person, not just the symptoms.

Help for itchy spots: Dab diluted cider vinegar or bicarbonate of soda on very itchy spots (1 tablespoon to 1 pint/½ liter of water), or let a not very sick child soak in a tepid bath to which a cup of vinegar or a handful of bicarbonate of soda has been added. Or blend a cup of dry oatmeal until fine and put a handful in the bath.

Help for sore eyes: Bathe eyes with Euphrasia (eyebright) lotion to ease soreness (a tablespoon to a pint of freshly boiled water; let it cool, strain it, and bathe eyes with a separate cotton ball for each eye).

Dosage: Give 1 tablet (of the 6C or 30C potency) every 2 hours for up to 6 doses, then 3 times daily once it has started to help. Tablets can be chewed or added to a small glass of water.

Stop once symptoms are considerably better.

Change the remedy after a day if there is no improvement or it has stopped helping.

Aromatherapy and Childhood Diseases
By Christa Obuchowski

Christa Obuchowski is a certified aromatherapist who received her training in Europe and the US. Her business, Body Therapy, is devoted to a full-spectrum approach, a holistic view of healing. She teaches aromatherapy at the New Mexico Academy of Healing Arts in Santa Fe, New Mexico. "Aromatherapy and Childhood Diseases" first appeared in Mothering, *no. 77 (Winter 1995).*

Aromatherapy can be a soothing, healing addition to your child's sickroom. The scents alone can lift the spirits of parents and children alike, as well as hasten the healing process. Current research has proven that essential oils have remarkable medicinal qualities. Distilled from the flowers, bark, roots, and leaves of plants, essential oils are antiviral, antibacterial, and antifungal. Certain plants, including lemon, thyme, rosemary, eucalyptus, peppermint, and German chamomile, possess antiseptic properties, which inhibit the development of *Staphylococcus*. Parents can easily learn a few simple steps to prevent the spread of germs, soothe and calm a cranky child, and reduce the discomfort of itching. In the formulas included here, three methods for using the essential oils are recommended: a room diffuser, sponge baths, and a massage formula.

General Guidelines
• If possible, select organic or wildcrafted oils of the best quality.
• Do not use essential oils on babies under three months old. With children under 18 months, use oils cautiously.
•For children ages 18 months to five years, double the base oil in massage formulas. (Diffuser and inhalation formulas do not need to be changed.)
•For children ages five to 15 years, use the full essential oil formula.
•Test for skin sensitivity by applying the oil formula to a small area of skin and then waiting a few minutes to see if there's a reaction. Also test to see if your child likes a scent before diffusing it. If he or she does not like the scent, do not diffuse it. Please keep essential oil bottles out of reach of children.
•Keep in mind that 1 ml is equal to 30 drops of oil; thus a 5-ml bottle of any oil will contain 150 drops.

Seek help from a certified aromatherapist if you have any questions or concerns regarding the use of oils on your child, especially if he or she has asthma, high or low blood pressure, is on chemotherapy, or has eczema or hypersensitive skin. If you are pregnant, consult an aromatherapist about which oils you may use safely during your pregnancy.

BASE OIL

This mixture makes a great base oil, but almond oil and grape seed oil work perfectly well by themselves as a base.

½ounce almond oil
½ounce jojoba oil
5 drops vitamin E oil (as an antioxidant)

AIR PURIFICATION FORMULA

Chickenpox, measles, mumps, scarlet fever, and whooping cough are all highly contagious illnesses. Use a room diffuser in the sickroom as well as in other parts of the home to cut down the spread of airborne germs. Diffusers act to distribute the essential oil molecules into the air. They come in many different forms, from those activated by candles to lightbulb rings. For a child's room, it's best to use an electrically generated fan unit since it will be quiet and can be left operating for long periods of time. The following formulas can be made up in large quantity, particularly since an illness may go on for weeks.

PURIFICATION 1

10 drops eucalyptus oil
  (*Eucalyptus radiata* or *Eucalyptus globulus*)
10 drops niaouli or tea tree oil
  (*Melaleuca qi. viridiflora*)
10 drops lavender (*Lavender vera*)

PURIFICATION 2

5 drops thyme oil (*Thyme linalol*)
10 drops lemon oil (*Citrus limonum*)
10 drops rosemary verbenone (*Rosmarinus officinalis*)

Blend these oils together. Shake well and use 3 drops in the diffuser

3 times daily. Lemon oil by itself is wonderfully refreshing for house purification.

SPONGE BATH OR ATOMIZER FORMULA

In treating chickenpox, it's most important to calm the irritating itching. Not only will this prevent scarring, it will also soothe nervous irritation. If your child cannot bear to be touched, use the atomizer in place of the sponge bath. Make this formula in a large quantity so that it can be used repeatedly. Distilled water is fine to use as a base, but floral water from a reputable company—either lavender, rose, eucalyptus, or chamomile—provides powerful therapeutic agents that will enhance the healing aspect of this formula. Floral waters are commonly available in local health food stores. Use them undiluted as a base in place of the plain water base. Floral waters are extremely gentle; even children with hypersensitive skin are able to use genuine floral waters without reaction. Floral waters can also be used by themselves.

6 ounces distilled or floral water
10 drops lavender oil (*Lavender vera*)
5 drops tea tree oil   (*Melaleuca alternifolia*)
5 drops German chamomile oil (*Matricariea recutita*)
2 drops peppermint oil (*Menta piperita*)

Blend these oils together with the floral water. The formula is ready to use immediately. Shake well before each application. Use soft, clean cloths to sponge the formula onto the child's rash or use the spray atomizer. Apply 3 times a day. If the child is well enough to tolerate a bath in the tub, add 2 drops lavender, 2 drops German chamomile, and 1 cup of bicarbonate of soda to the bathwater. When itching is extreme, dip a cotton swab into pure lavender oil (*Lavender vera*) and apply to the breakout.

CALMING REST FORMULA

When children are ill, it's difficult for them to get the rest and relaxation that is so beneficial to their healing process. Make this formula up in quantity for naptime as well as bedtime.

15 drops lavender oil (*Lavender vera*)

10 drops Mandarin red oil (*Citrus reticulata*)
5 drops Roman chamomile oil (*Chamaemelum nobile*)

Blend these essential oils together and use 4 drops in the diffuser at naptime and at bedtime.

BREATHE EASY FORMULA

Whooping cough is quite a serious illness and can keep both child and parent up for weeks. This formula is designed to alleviate difficult breathing and calm the bronchi.

FORMULA 1

10 drops eucalyptus oil (*Eucalyptus globulus*)
10 drops lavender oil (*Lavender vera*)
7 drops hyssop oil (*Hyssopus off. decumbens*)
3 drops thyme linalol oil (*Thymus vulg. linalol sweet*)

FORMULA 2

10 drops niaouli oil (*Melaleuca qi. viridiflora*)
10 drops myrtle oil (*Myrtus communis*)
5 drops cypress oil (*Cupressus sempervirens*)
3 drops thyme linalol oil (*Thymus vulg. linalol sweet*)

Blend the essential oils together and add 4 drops to a diffuser or a hot-air vaporizer. Keep the child's room as humid as possible to avoid dehydration of the bronchial tract.

HELPING HAND MASSAGE OIL FORMULA

Every childhood illness brings with it aches and pains. Mumps and whooping cough can leave your child tired, restless, and out of sorts. A light massage can convey love and tenderness, as well as relax sore muscles. Make this formula up in quantity and keep it on hand during your child's confinement.

1 ounce base oil (see formula above)
4 drops lavender oil (*Lavender vera*)
2 drops German chamomile oil (*Matricaria recutita*)
2 drops everlasting oil (*Helichrysum italicum*)

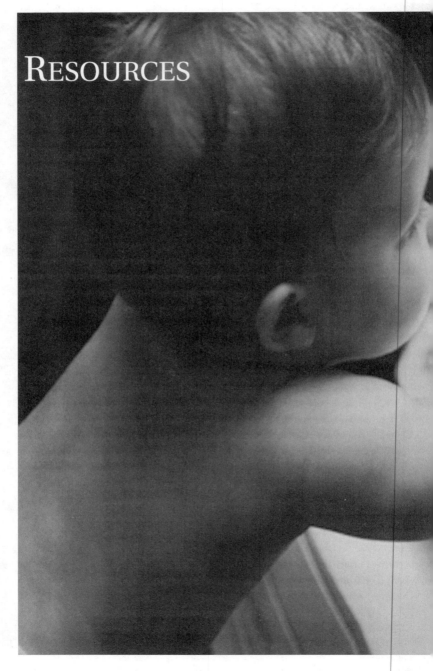

RESOURCES

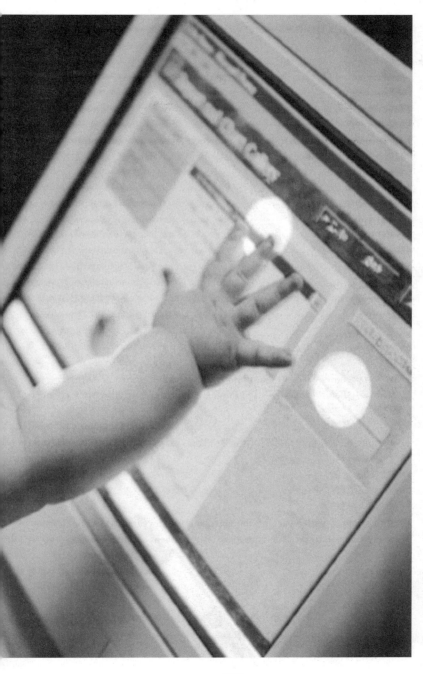

GENERAL RESOURCES

American Natural Hygiene Society
James Michael Lennon, Executive director
PO Box 30630
Tampa, FL 33630
813-855-6607
This group empowers families to create high-level health and compassionate awareness through "living in harmony with nature."

Barge Chiropractic Clinic S. C.
322 Cameron Ave.
La Crosse, WI 54601
1-800-882-5470
608-784-3279 (fax)
Free brochure written by Dr. Barge.

Citizens for the Repeal of the Vaccination Laws
Walene James
2101 Pallets Ct.
Virginia Beach, VA 23454
757-486-3129
Has comprehensive, up-to-date information. Author of *Immunization: The Reality Behind the Myth* (see Publications). $5.00 for introductory packet.

Determined Parents to Stop Hurting Our Tots (DPTSHOT)
Marge Grant
915 S. University Ave.
Beaverdam, WI 53916
414-887-1133
Marge has lived with a vaccine-damaged son for 35 years and has been actively involved in vaccine issues. She is available as a contact person.

Hahnemann Pharmacy
828 San Pablo Ave.
Albany, CA 94706
510-527-3003 or 1-888-427-6422
Specializes in homeopathic remedies, many of which are made on the

premises. *The Immunization Decision* by Randall Neustaedter is available directly from the pharmacy for $8.95 plus $5.00 shipping/handling (if prepaid).

Homeopathic Educational Services
2124 Kittredge St.
Berkeley, CA 94704
510-649-0294
1-800-359-9051

Humanitarian Publishing Co.
PO Box 220
Quakertown, PA 18951
1-800-300-5168
Has books available on vaccinations by R. S. Clymer, MD, Dr. G. E. Poesnecker, and Harold Buttram, MD. Prices range from $4.00 to $14.00.

Dr. Daniel Lander
Family Chiropractor
RR1, Box 1106
Coopers Mills, ME 04341
Send an SASE to receive Dr. Lander's pamphlet *On Immunizations*. An updated version of his 1980 book, *Chiropractic and Wholistic Health*, is still in the works and should be available in 1996 for $4.95.

National Vaccine Information Center (NVIC)
Dissatisfied Parents Together (DPT)
512 W. Maple Ave., Ste. 206
Vienna, VA 22180
1-800-909-SHOT
703-938-DPT3
703-938-5768 (fax)
A national nonprofit educational organization representing parents and healthcare professionals concerned about childhood diseases and side effects of vaccines. The center provides support to help educate parents about vaccine safety and their right to choose immunizations, as well as support for parents and families who have experienced a vaccine reaction. *The Vaccine Reaction* is a bimonthly newsletter for $18.00/year. Other available publications include *Vaccination: A Guide for Parents*

($7.00), *Whooping Cough: The DPT Vaccine and Reducing Reactions* ($8.00), *A Shot in the Dark* ($15.45), *The Consumer's Guide to Childhood Vaccinations* ($9.00 plus $2.00 shipping), plus videotapes, lists of problem DPT lots, and other books on the vaccination controversy.

National Vaccine Injury Compensation Program
Health Resources and Services Administration
Parklawn Bldg., Room 8A-35
5600 Fishers Ln.
Rockville, MD 20857
1-800-338-2382
Administered by the Department of Health and Human Services to provide payments for persons who have died or suffered an injury associated with vaccines for DPT, measles, mumps, and rubella, as well as oral and inactivated polio vaccine, Hib, hepatitis, varicella.

Natural Immunity Information Network
PO Box 20723
New York, NY 10009
212-978-8789
Publishes newsletter, $5.00/year. Offers local community-based support in NYC area.

Vaccine Information and Awareness (VIA)
Karin Schumacher
12799 La Tortola
San Diego, CA 92129
619-484-3197
Fax 619-484-1187
E-mail: via@access1.net
Website: www.access1.net/via

Benjamin Russell Council for Economic Inquiry
224 Fulbright Dr.
Mountain Home, AR 72653-8709
501-492-5743
Benjamin Russell has been teaching students how to get well and stay well by following a way of life called "natural hygiene." He has reprints of articles on vaccinations, drugs, and medications. Send $5.00 plus an SASE

for information.

Rutherford Institute
PO Box 7482
Charlottesville, VA 22906
804-978-3888
Provides legal brief on compulsory vaccinations on state-to-state basis. Advocates on issues of religious liberty and offers advice on finding legal assistance in any area regarding religious freedom.

Vaccine Research Institute
PO Box 4182
Northbrook, IL 60065
847-564-1403
Josephine Szczesny
Publishes a reference list for $4.00 of scientific articles citing adverse reactions to vaccinations. Also an immunization binder, *"Yes" or "No,"* for $35.00.

The Bell of Atri, Inc.
J. Anthony Morris
23-E Ridge Rd.
Greenbelt, MD 20770
301-474-5031

STATE ORGANIZATIONS

Citizens for Healthcare Freedom
PO Box 62282
Durham, NC 27715
919-859-3321
919-383-1000
E-mail: aphillip@emal.unc.edu

Massachusetts Citizens for Vaccination Choice(MCVC)
PO Box 1033
East Arlington, MA 02174-0020
617-646-4797
E-mail: MCVCHQ@juno.com

Michigan Opposing Mandatory Vaccines
PO Box 1121
Troy, MI 48099-1121
810-447-2418

Missouri Citizens' Coalition for Freedom in Health Care
PO Box 190318
St. Louis, MO 63119-0318
314-968-8755

Ohio Parents for Vaccine Safety
Kristine Severyn, RPh, PhD
251 W. Ridgeway Dr.
Dayton, OH 45459
937-435-4750
Has a national quarterly newsletter and resource material. Send SASE for free general information packet.

LAWYERS AND INFORMATION ON THE LAW

Association of Trial Lawyers (ATLA)
1050 31st St. N.W.
Washington, DC 20007
202-965-3500
Provides information regarding attorneys with experience in vaccine injury litigation.

Kirkpatrick Dilling
150 N. Wacker, Ste. 1242
Chicago, IL 60606
312-236-8417
Legal health rights defender.

Andrew Dodd
21515 Hawthorne Blvd., #840
Torrance, CA 90503
310-316-6223
Attorney for safe vaccines and help with exemption requirements.

Bonnie Plumeri Franz
815 Knox St.
Ogdensburg, NY 13669
315-393-2950
Lobbies government for vaccine laws and exemptions. Keeps very up-to-date on legislation. She has published letters in *Mothering*.

Melvin Kimmel
227 Corbin Pl.
Brooklyn, NY 11235-4901
718-648-2161
Attorney for safe vaccines.

Sharon Kimmelman
Vaccination Alternatives
The Right to Know, The Freedom to Abstain
PO Box 346
New York, NY 10023
212-873-5051
Twelve years experience, literature, counseling, advocacy, and parent networks. Introductory packet $5.00 plus SASE.

Walter Kyle
60 South St
Hingham, MA 02043
508-747-5522
FAX: 508-747-5533
An Attorney in private practice. Kyle is an expert on vaccine product liability and the manufacturing of polio vaccines. His article linking HIV with polio vaccines appeared in *The Lancet*, Vol. 339: March 7, 1992.

Kirk A. McCarville
2400 E. Arizona
Biltmore Circle, Ste 1430
Phoenix, AZ 85016
602-468-1714
Attorney who represents vaccine-injured children; may be willing to testify in cases involving decision not to vaccinate.

Peter H. Meyers
2000 G Street NW, Suite 200
Washington, DC 20052
202-994-7463
Fax: 202-994-4946

Peter H. Meyers, JD, is Professor of clinical law and director of the Vaccine Injury Project, George Washington University Law School. Meyers supervises law students who represent individuals seeking financial compensation before the US Court of Federal Claims under the National Childhood Vaccine Injury Act of 1986.

INFORMATION ON VACCINE INJURY

National Vaccine Information Center (NVIC)
Dissatisfied Parents Together (DPT)
512 W. Maple Ave., Ste. 206
Vienna, VA 22180
1-800-909-SHOT
703-938-DPT3
703-938-5768 (fax)

A national nonprofit educational organization representing parents and healthcare professionals concerned about childhood diseases and side effects of vaccines. The center provides support to help educate parents about vaccine safety and their right to choose immunizations, as well as support for parents and families who have experienced a vaccine reaction. *The Vaccine Reaction* is a bimonthly newsletter for $18.00/year. Other available publications include *Vaccination: A Guide for Parents* ($7.00), *Whooping Cough: The DPT Vaccine and Reducing Reactions* ($8.00), *A Shot in the Dark* ($15.45), *The Consumer's Guide to Childhood Vaccinations* ($9.00 plus $2.00 shipping), plus videotapes, lists of problem DPT lots, and other books on the vaccination controversy.

National Vaccine Injury Compensation Program
Health Resources and Services Administration
Parklawn Bldg., Room 8A-35
5600 Fishers Ln.
Rockville, MD 20857
1-800-338-2382

Administered by the Department of Health and Human Services to provide payments for persons who have died or suffered an injury associated with vaccines for DPT, measles, mumps, and rubella, as well as oral and inactivated polio vaccine.

Philip Incao, MD
Anthroposophic and Homeopathic Medicine
Steiner Medical Associates
Gilpin Street Holistic Center
1624 Gilpin St.
Denver, CO 80218
303-323-2100
Fax: 303-321-3737

Arno Brunier, DC
108 Latigo Rd.
Durango, CO 81301
970-247-0004

Amy Rothenberg, ND
Paul Herscu, ND
115 Elm St.
Enfield, CT 06083
860-763-1225

Autism/Intolerance/Allergy Network
AIA-USA
127 East Main St, Rm 106
Riverhead, NY 11901
516-369-9340

Autism Research Institute
4182 Adams Ave.
San Diego, CA 92116
619-281-7175
Developmental Delay Registry
Patricia Lemer, MEd NCC
6701 Fairfax Rd.
Chevy Chase, MD 20185
301-652-2263

Feingold Association of the United States
PO Box 6550
Alexandria, VA 22306
703-768-FAUS (3287)

Carbon Based Corporation
Patricia Kane, PhD
920 Incline Way, Ste 2C
Incline Village, NV 89451
702-832-8485
Fax: 702-832-8488

The American Holistic Medical Association
4101 Lake Boone Trail, #201
Raleigh, NC 27606
919-787-5181
Send $5.00 for list of practitioners.

World Chiropractic Alliance
2950 N. Dobson Rd. Ste. 1
Chandler, AZ 85224
800-347-1011

International Chiropractors Association
1110 N. Glebe Rd. Ste. 1000
Arlington, VA 22201
703-528-5000

International Chiropractic Pediatric Association
414 Ponce de Leon Ave.
Atlanta, GA 30308
404-872-5437

National Center for Homeopathy
801 N. Fairfax, Ste 306
Alexandria, VA 22314
703-548-7790
Send $5.00 for list of practitioners.

American Association of Oriental Medicine

433 Front St.
Catasauqua, PA 18032
610-433-2448

American Association of Naturopathic Physicians
2366 Eastlake Ave. E #322
Seattle, WA 98102
206-323-7610
Send $5 for list of practitioners.

Vaccine Adverse Effect Reporting System
Department of Health and Human Services
PO Box 1100
Rockville, MD 20849-111
1-800-822-7967

PUBLICATIONS

The Case Against Immunizations
Richard Moskowitz, MD
173 Mt. Auburn St.
Watertown, MA 02172
617-923-4604
Reprints of lectures on vaccinations given by Moskowitz available for $3.00.

DPT: A Shot in the Dark
Harris L. Coulter and Barbara Loe Fisher
Harcourt Brace Jovanovich
1985, 1991
$15.45
The Consumer's Guide to Childhood Vaccinations, Barbara Love Fisher ($9.00 plus $2.00 shipping), available directly from the National Vaccine Information Center/DPT, 512 W. Maple Ave., Ste. 206, Vienna, VA 22180. 703-938-DPT3.

Epidemiology and Prevention of Vaccine Preventable Diseases
William Atkinson et al., eds.

2nd edition, 1995
Department of Health and Human Services and Centers for Disease Control and Prevention
Order by calling 404-639-3534.

The Immunization Resource Guide
Diane Rozario
Patter Publications
PO Box 204
Burlington, IA 52601-0204
319-752-0039
319-754-7970 (fax)
Newly revised in 1997, 3rd edition
$11.95 ppd.
A thorough guide, including reviews of available books, health and vaccine organizations, and vaccine product information.

What Every Parent Should Know About Childhood Immunizations
Jamie Murphy
1997
International Chiropractic Association
$13.95 plus $300 shipping and handling
800-423-4690
703-528-5000

*Immunization: Theory vs. Reality
Neil Z. Miller
New Atlantean Press
1995
$12.95 plus $3.50 s/h
Exposé on vaccinations, including medical ploys, Gulf War syndrome, government coercion, and personal stories.
Immunization: The Reality Behind the Myth
Walene James
Bergin & Garvey
1995 (revised)
(check local bookstore)

Mother to Mother

PO Box 1029-198
Van Nuys, CA 91408
818-989-7707
Newletter, $14.95/four issues. Back issues on vaccinations available.

Out of Silence: A Journey into Language
Russell Martin
Henry Holt
1994 (out of print)
Story of an 18-month-old boy damaged by the pertussis vaccine who developed autism.

Pure Water Gazette
PO Box 2783
Denton, TX 76202
817-382-3814
Back articles on vaccinations available free.

Second Opinion Newsletter
PO Box 467939
Atlanta, GA 31146
800-728-2288
Publishes monthly newsletter on alternative remedies, $39.00/yr., and *Immunizations: The Terrible Risks Your Children Face*, 1993, $12.00.

*Vaccination: 100 Years of Orthodox Research Shows that Vaccines Represent a Medical Assault on the Immune System
Viera Scheibner
The Australian Print Group, Maryborough, Victoria, Australia
1993
$26.95 plus $3.50 s/h
Available in North America from New Atlantean Press.

‡*Vaccination, Social Violence & Criminality:*
The Medical Assault on the American Brain
Harris L. Coulter
1990
$25.00 hardcover, $14.95 paperback
‡*The Vaccine Guide*

Randall Neustaedter
1996
$12.95
‡Both available from:
North Atlantic Books
PO Box 12327
Berkeley, CA 94712
1-800-337-2665
Also, *The Immunization Decision* is available from Homeopathic Educational Services and Hahnemann Pharmacy (see General Resources).

"The Vaccine Machine"
1000 Wilson Blvd.
Arlington, VA 22229
703-276-5800
Send a SASE for this article, which is an exposé on vaccinations by the Gannett News Service.

Vaccines
Stanley Plotkin and Edward Mortimer
Philadelphia
W. B. Saunders
1994, 2nd edition
$179.00
1-800-545-2522

*Vaccines: Are They Really Safe and Effective? A Parent's Guide to Childhood Shots
Neil Z. Miller
New Atlantean Press
1996, updated 6th edition
$8.95 plus $3.50 s/h.
PO Box 9638-16
Santa Fe, NM 87504
505-983-1856
Evaluates "mandated" vaccines to determine their safety, effectiveness, long-term effects, and the cause of decline in each disease. 80 pages, 12 charts, more than 300 citations.

What about Immunization? Exposing the Vaccine Philosophy
Cynthia Cournoyer
Clear Communications
1995, 6th edition
7185 Redwood Highway
Grants Pass, OR 97527
541-474-7886
$15.49 ppd.

What Doctors Don't Tell You Newsletter
and *Mother Knows Best* Newsletter
4 Wallace Road
London N1 2PG
ENGLAND
44+171-354-4592
Founder Lynne McTaggart authored "The MMR Vaccine" published in *Mothering,* Spring 1992. *What Doctors Don't Tell You,* £29.95/year plus £6 for overseas postage. Visa/MC accepted, or check/money order in British pounds sterling only.

Your Personal Guide to Immunization Exemptions
Grace Girdwain
8320 S. Nashville Ave.
Burbank, IL 60459
Exemption guide available for $10.95.

"Vaccination Dangers," Andrea Rock, *Money Magazine*
December 1996
Volume 25, Number 12
PO Box 60001
Tampa, FL 33660
212-522-5454

Travel Information and International Contacts

Aurum Healing Centre
PO Box 155
Daylesford 3460
AUSTRALIA
(05)239225

Publishes *Vaccination? A Review of Risks and Alternatives*, 5th edition. Includes a specific homeopathic program for protection from common childhood diseases as an alternative to vaccination, and a supplementary homeopathic program if your child is exposed to infection. A$3.00 surface, A$8.00 airmail as an Australian bank draft.

Vaccination Awareness and Information Service
PO Box 9086
Manly West, QLD 4179
AUSTRALIA
07-8008821 or 07-8932323
07-8932423 (fax)
Offers a free pamphlet as well as a newsletter for $10.00/yr. and audiotapes. Vaccination Information Network Qld, Inc. (VINE)
P O Box 808
Nambour, QLD 4560
AUSTRALIA
61-74-48-4136 or 49-1177
Books and a newsletter available. Membership is $20.00.

Infor Vie Saine ASBL
143, P. Babin
B-5020- Malonne
BELGIUM
3281-445283
Puts out a pamphlet with statements by Dr. Mendelsohn (not published in English).

Canadian Natural Health Association
439 Wellington St. W., Unit 5
Toronto, Ontario M5V 1E7
CANADA
416-977-2642
416-280-6025 information line
If you live in Canada, this group will be able to direct your questions on vaccinations.

International Association for Medical Assistance to Travellers (IAMAT)
417 Center St.
Lewiston, NY 14092

716-754-4883
Canadian Office:
40 Regal Rd.
Guelph, Ontario N1K 1B5
CANADA
519-836-0102
This association is very helpful when you are traveling and has information on international vaccine laws and traveling requirements.

Edda West
Vaccine Education, Research, and Alternatives
814 Shaw St.
Toronto, Ontario M6G 3M1
CANADA
416-534-1477

Association for Vaccine Damaged Children
67 Shier
Winnipeg, Manitoba R3R 2H2
CANADA
204-895-9192
Support group started by parents whose children either died from or were injured by vaccinations.

Primal Health Research
59 Roderick Rd.
London NW3 2NP
ENGLAND
44 +171-2675123 (fax)
Michel Odent's newsletter, containing information on vaccinations. $18.00/yr.

The Informed Parent
19 Woodlands Rd.
Harrow, Middlesex HA1 2RT
ENGLAND
44+181-8611022 (tel. & fax)
A group that promotes awareness, understanding, and support for parents regardless of their decision. Has a newsletter and list of books and videos available.

Association of Parents of Vaccine Damaged Children
2 Church St.
Shipston on Stour
Warwickshire CV36 4AP
ENGLAND
Rosemary Fox
44+1608-661595
Formed in 1973 to press the British government to set up a compensation fund for children injured by vaccinations.

Lynne McTaggart
4 Wallace Rd.
London N1 2PG
ENGLAND
44+171-354-4592
Authored "The MMR Vaccine," published in *Mothering,* Spring 1992. Publishes newsletters *What Doctors Don't Tell You* and *Mother Knows Best* (see Publications section for subscription details).

Immunization Awareness Society of Finland
Box 217
SF-01300 Vantaa
FINLAND
Yves Delatte
Delatte has written a book called *Vaccinations: The Untold Truth,* and she accepts donations. All her material has been derived from official medical sources.

Association Liberté Information Santé
19 rue de l'Argentiere
63200 Riom
FRANCE
33-73630221
Sends a quarterly review to its members and has published a book on hepatitis. The group supports freedom of choice.

Dr. Gerhard Buchwald
Obersteben, Am Wolfsbuhl 28
95138 Bad Steben
GERMANY

49-92888328

Has a considerable amount of information available. In the near future he will publish a book that will be translated into English.

Nederlandse Vereniging Kritisch Prikken
Leutherhoekweg 25
6171 RW Stein
THE NETHERLANDS
0031-46337859 (phone and fax)
0031-464337859 (after 10/10/95)
Information is available, but not in English.

The Immunisation Awareness Society, Inc.
PO Box 56-048
Dominion Rd.
Auckland
NEW ZEALAND
Formed in 1988 to ensure that all parents have sufficient information to enable them to make an informed choice about vaccination. The society believes that people can only give informed consent to this medical procedure if they have access to all the information available, for and against vaccination. Subscription available for NZ$30.00/yr.

Groupe Medical de Reflexion
sur le Vaccin R O R
Case postale
1010 Lausanne
SWITZERLAND
031-301-26-50

Aerzte-Arbeitsgruppe fur
differenziert MMR-IMPFUNGEN
3000 Berne
SWITZERLAND
A group of doctors who object to the compulsory MMR campaign (using the US as a model example) and are informing others of the cons of the MMR vaccine. "The doctors who belong to the two working groups were not, as a whole, opposed to the principle of the vaccine itself. They advocate, however, a detailed vaccination practice, decided on an individual basis, which would consider the problems associated with each of the three dis-

eases separately. They support an approach that does not fundamentally alter the epidemiology of these three diseases, while respecting the freedom of choice of the parents."

These resources are current as of June 1997.

STATE EXEMPTIONS

BASIC INFORMATION

Some schools accept medical exemptions, such as a letter from the child's pediatrician. Talk to your doctor. Perhaps he or she can find a medical reason why your child should not be immunized. Maybe the doctor can, in all good conscience, certify that your child has received all the vaccinations that you both agree are necessary.

Send a letter to the school authorities stating that you reject vaccinations for personal reasons or on constitutional grounds. Some states have this loophole written into their school codes.

You probably know whether your own religion prohibits vaccinations. If not, this is an issue you may wish to discuss with your own clergy or those of other religions. Some people have gone so far as to form their own religion, whose major tenet is prohibition of vaccinations.

Bring political pressure to bear on your elected representatives to amend compulsory vaccination statutes.

Consult an attorney to decide on possible legal action.

(Adapted from Robert Mendelson, MD, *The People's Doctor* 4, no. 5).

THESE RESOURCES ARE CURRENT AS OF 1997.

STATE EXEMPTION INFORMATION

Do you know your state exemptions? If not, you may obtain a copy of compulsory vaccination regulations in your state by contacting the State Health and Environment Department, Division of Public Health. This may be called something different in each state. You will find the correct title, address, and phone number in the state section of the blue pages in your local telephone book. This information can also be found through the local county health department or the public library. You have the legal right to see the information in full. No one will be interrogated about vaccination beliefs simply for requesting the information.

Currently, each state allows some kind of exemption from vaccination. This differs state by state. For instance, in New Mexico we have "Religious/Conscientious Objection to Immunization." Many states have religious exemption, in which a parent is required to be a bona fide member of a specific religious group that objects to vaccination. Here in New Mexico we can be exempt because of our "individual religious beliefs." We must fill out a form, sign it in the presence of a notary public, and return it to the State Health and Environment Department (HED) for authorization. The form is then sent directly to the school, daycare, or camp, and to the child's parents. In New Mexico the exemption form must be completed and renewed at the beginning of each school year.

Susan Mansbach, a *Mothering* reader, suggests using the following words in a letter to the school/state board. They worked for her:

"In accordance with GS 130A-157 *(substitute appropriate state law)*, under the title "Religious Exemption," I hereby declare that as a parent having responsibility for *(child's name)*, a minor enrolled in *(name of school)*, I request that the said minor be exempt from said vaccinations on grounds that administration of the immunizing agents conflicts with our religious tenets and practices."

Alabama..334-293-6448
    Medical, religious, philosophical

Alaska 907-465-3353
    Medical, religious

Arizona 602-506-6767
    Medical, religious, philosophical
    (philosophical is not accepted in preschool)

Arkansas 501-661-2000
    Medical, religious

California...415-554-2830
    Religious, medical, philosophical

Colorado..303-692-2000
    Religious, medical, philosophical

Connecticut..203-566-5657
    Medical, religious

Delaware..302-739-4746
    Medical, religious (must be notarized)

Florida 904-487-3186
    Medical, religious

Georgia 404-657-3158
    Medical, religious

Hawaii...808-733-9220
    Medical, religious, philosophical

Idaho..208-334-5945
    Medical, religious, philosophical

Illinois..217-785-2033
    Medical, religious

Indiana 317-383-6100
    Medical, religious

Iowa..515-281-7993
    Medical, religious

Kansas..913-296-1500
    Medical, religious

Kentucky..502-564-3970
    Medical, religious

Louisiana...504-483-1900
    Medical, religious, philosophical

Maine..207-287-3746
    Medical, religious, philosophical

Maryland 410-225-6679
    Medical, religious

Massachusetts..617-983-6800
    Medical, religious, philosophical

Michigan...517-335-8159
    Medical, religious, philosophical

Minnesota 612-623-5237
    Medical, religious, philosophical

Mississippi...601-364-2666
    Medical

Missouri..314-751-6400
    Medical, religious

Montana 406-444-2544
    Medical, religious

Nebraska..402-471-2133
    Medical, religious, philosophical
    (must be notarized)

Nevada...702-687-4800
    Medical, religious

New Hampshire...603-271-4482
    Medical, religious, philosophical
    (must be notarized)

New Jersey...609-588-7512
or 800-367-6543 (local)
    Medical, religious

New Mexico..505-827-2369
    Medical, religious, philosophical

New York..212-349-2664
    Medical, religious

North Carolina...919-733-7752
    Medical, religious

North Dakota...701-328-2378
    Medical, religious, philosophical

Ohio...614-466-0249
    Medical, religious, philosophical

Oklahoma...405-271-5600
    Medical, religious, philosophical

Oregon...503-731-4020
    Medical, religious

Pennsylvania...215-685-6740
    Medical, religious, philosophical

Rhode Island 401-277-2577
    Medical, religious

South Carolina 803-737-4160
    Medical, religious (must be notarized)

South Dakota 605-733-3361
    Medical, religious, philosophical

Tennessee 901-576-7600
    Medical, religious

Texas 512-458-7284
    Medical, religious

Utah 801-538-9450
    Medical, religious, philosophical

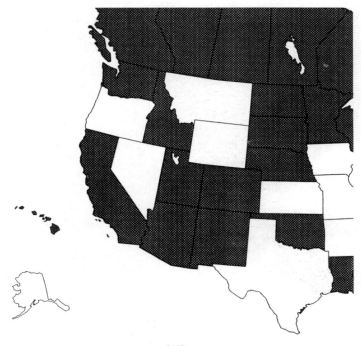

Vermont..802-863-7638
    Medical, religious, philosophical

Virginia 804-786-6246
    Medical, religious

Washington 360-753-3495
    Medical, religious, philosophical

Washington, DC..202-576-7130
    Medical, religious

West Virginia 304-558-2188
    Medical

Wisconsin...715-836-2499
    Medical, religious, philosophical

Wyoming 307-777-7952
    Medical, religious

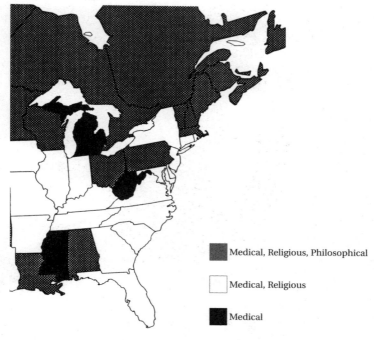

Medical, Religious, Philosophical

Medical, Religious

Medical